Becky 3/80

TISSUE CLEANSING THROUGH BOWEL MANAGEMENT

FROM THE SIMPLE TO THE ULTIMATE

by Dr. Bernard Jensen, D.C.

Coauthored with Sylvia Bell

THE INFORMATION IN THIS BOOK IS A GATHERING OF KNOWLEDGE FROM MANY CORNERS OF THE WORLD AND FROM CONSIDERABLE SANITARIUM EXPERIENCE. IN ADDITION, IT REPRESENTS A SYNTHESIS OF THE STUDIES AND EXPERIENCES OF MANY INDIVIDUALS WHO HAVE RESEARCHED THE ART OF CLEANLINESS FROM THE INSIDE OUT.

10th Edition
(Over 100,000 Copies Sold)

Cover design by Debra Diogo

Published by
Bernard Jensen Enterprises
24360 Old Wagon Road
Escondido, California 92027

DEDICATION

This book is dedicated to those who want to take the higher path, which is the one approved by God, and to those who would be free and cleansed of the old so as to embrace the coming into the new and higher life.

"Cleanse and purify thyself and I will exalt thee to the throne of power."

"Be thou clean."

The results obtained with the program outlined in this book should command the interest of every physician who claims to follow a preventive health care philosophy. It is a powerful tool when used to overcome the entrenched effects of chronic diseases, as are an estimated 80% of those found in this country. It is a most ideal way to turn such conditions around toward rejuvenation and well-being.

CONTENTS

FOREWORD

Publishing this book has been somewhat difficult due to the nature of the subject matter. Bowel management is virtually an undiscussed topic in our culture and Western society. It's not nice to talk about. Somehow the unspoken idea has crept upon us which implies that the bowel will take care of itself. Also along with this erroneous belief comes another which implies that anything we may buy in the supermarket or prepare in our kitchen will be received with gratitude by the gastro-intestinal system. Dr. Tom Spies, recipient of the American Medical Association's Distinguished Service Award has said, "All the chemicals used in the body—except for the oxygen we breathe and the water we drink—are taken in through food."

Unfortunately, the selection of poor foods and improper preparation methods often lead to bowel problems. Specifically, researchers have shown that regular use of refined carbohydrates and a lack of fiber in the diet increase the transit time of bowel wastes and stimulate production of putrefactive bacteria in the bowel. Both of these factors have been linked not only to bowel diseases such as colitis, diverticulosis and cancer but also to chronic disease elsewhere in the body.

Fortunately, what medical scientists call the "irritable bowel syndrome" can be prevented or reversed in most cases by following the program described in this book. There are methods, however, such as proper diet, which will lead to the same results but over a longer period of time.

The response to the first edition of this book has been wonderful. We have received many suggestions and comments which have led us to make revisions and additions to make this book more responsive to your needs.

It often takes an act of resolution and courage in order to get out of the bowel situation in which so many people find themselves. There is no better way than taking positive, affirmative action. The instructions given in this book will give you the opportunity to take greater responsibility over your level of health and well-being. Improving the condition of your bowel will give you worthwhile dividends in renewed health, energy and vitality, an investment well made.

The program outlined in this book is just the beginning of a new path. Once the bowel is cleansed of accumulated waste material, the next step begins. Giving up old habits is a very difficult thing for most

1

people but is absolutely essential to regaining full health. The building process begins when correct, life-giving attitudes and habits take over. We can regenerate the body when we have clean tissues that are able to draw all the nutrients and chemical elements we need from the foods we eat. Coffee and donuts will not do the job; sugar and white bread won't either. If old habits are not given up, only temporary "flash" results will be experienced.

This book has been made available for the person who wants to take greater responsibility for his or her own health and well-being. The 7-day cleansing program described here has been used by many in their own homes with safety.

Rome was not built in a day, nor are the dividends of effective bowel management always evident right away. It can take months or even years to correct problems that have taken many years to come about. Developing proper elimination is half the job. The other half is rebuilding damaged tissue.

CAUTION

I want to make clear that the program described in this book is not being represented as a cure for any disease or ailment. It is simply a method of cleaning out the bowel and of restoring regular bowel habits, which leads to a cleaner body through more efficient elimination of wastes.

The program described here will seldom conflict with any other therapy or treatment, but if you are under a doctor's care, it is best to discuss this program with him and seek his counsel and support. If your doctor is interested in natural and preventive health care, he will understand that a clean body is more responsive to any therapeutic measure he feels you need. Our program is not intended to supplant qualified professional health care.

Not everyone needs this program, and we are not recommending it as a universal panacea. But, there are many who will benefit from it.

We recommend that the seriously ill and the elderly go easy with this program, seeking the advice of their doctor in modifying any of its features to conform to their specific needs and limitations. We have attempted to make this book as complete and as clear as possible, to answer all potential questions and to avoid confusion. Questions and inquiries from professional practitioners are welcomed.

If you suffer from a bleeding bowel or any severe bowel disturbance, it is imperative that a doctor's supervision be employed.

Chapter 1

INTRODUCTION TO RAISING BOWEL CONSCIOUSNESS

TWO MIRACLES*

As out of dirty mud-beds, gorgeous lilies grow—
So out of bent-old-age, comes vibrant youth!
And youth from age, is not a greater miracle
than pure white lilies growing out of mud!

In the 50 years I've spent helping people to overcome illness, disability and disease, it has become crystal clear that poor bowel management lies at the root of most people's health problems.

In treating over 300,000 patients, it is the bowel that invariably has to be cared for first before any effective healing can take place.

In times past, knowledge of the bowel was more widespread and people were taught how to care for the bowel. Somehow bowel wisdom got lost and it became something that no one wanted to talk about anymore.

By putting the bowel in the closet and making believe it doesn't exist, many people have gone down the path of improper living, treating the bowel indiscriminately and reaping the sad harvest in later years.

Knowing the ways of keeping the bowel healthy and in good shape is the best way I know to keep away from the grip of disease and sickness.

The bowel-wise person is the one who is armed with good knowledge, practices discrimination in his eating habits and walks the path of the higher life. His days are blessed with health, vitality, optimism and the fulfillment of life's goals. He is a blessing and source of inspiration to family and associates. His cheerful disposition comes from having a vital, toxin-free body made possible by the efficient, regular and cleansing action of a loved and well-cared for bowel. Every person who desires the higher things in life must be aware of proper bowel management; what it is, how it works and what is required. In so doing, you will discover many secrets of life, develop a positive attitude toward yourself and become the master of body function.

*From *"Mysterious Catalytic Foods,"* by Brown Landone.

I believe autointoxication is currently the number one source of the misery and decay we are witnessing in our society and culture today. Through it comes the host of uncleanliness, with its entourage of imbalance, derangements, perversions, sickness and disease. Autointoxication becomes a powerful master over the body, robbing the inhabitant of clear thinking, discrimination, sound judgment, vitality, health, happiness and loved ones. Its rewards are disillusionment, bitterness, disappointment, financial chaos and failure.

Overcoming the effects of autointoxication can be a long and difficult task. It is much preferred to avoid it in the beginning than to have to struggle with the consequences in later life. I believe in educating not medicating.

The topic of bowel management is a broad one. Many books have been written on the subject. Many different views have been projected, and there is some confusion about exactly what constitutes proper bowel hygiene.

In this book, I give you the best information currently available and the accumulated wisdom gathered from a lifetime devoted to natural therapeutics as it relates to bowel care.

I've traveled to the farthest corners of the earth searching for the secrets to health and long life and want to share with you my discoveries so that all who will, may partake in the nurturing of these seeds and harvest the benefits of the higher life.

This is a book of experiences that should awaken a person to the realization that the greatest healing power comes from within out. We find that healing comes according to the one law that I have followed in my sanitarium work for years; that is *Hering's Law of Cure*. It states that *"All cure starts from within out and from the head down and in reverse order as the symptoms have appeared."*

This book takes into consideration one of the first things that has to be managed in our body maintenance program. No one has ever had a home nor any acreage to take care of in which they did not have to consider the elimination of waste.

Years ago it was found that many of man's diseases came from a lack of sanitation. People would let the urine and toxic material from the bowel just travel through the streets. This situation attracted many of the diseases that were so prevalent throughout the world at one time.

Sanitation has come about in many ways. Underground sewers take away potentially harmful wastes. Packaging of food has kept it sanitary. Boiling, scorching and burning have broken up bacterial effects that could be transferred to the body. We find, however, that to take care of eliminations properly, we must start in the very beginning to look after these things. We have to stop dumping waste indiscriminately. We must stop having unsanitary conditions and their effects flowing through our bodies.

We have a sanitation department in our body. We have a cesspool, a sewer, so to speak, and we must keep it clean. We must set it up bacterially-wise so that we do not get into the disharmony or disease conditions.

This book gives valuable information about the care of the body from the bowel elimination standpoint in particular. It has been my work to make sure that upon a patient's first visit, all the elimination channels are put in good working condition. To try to take care of any symptom in the body without a good elimination system is futile.

In order to explain this work, I will present to you just a little bit of the anatomy and physiology of the digestive and eliminative systems and some of the things that possibly many are not aware of because they are not generally talked about. The average person doesn't want to talk about the bowel, and is not sufficiently informed about this important function of life to avoid the consequences of ignorance in bowel management. But, it is time we come out and talk about this part of the body, which is so much in need of care in this day and age.

When we eat foods that are not whole, when they aren't raw or don't contain enough bulk, we are inviting trouble. When we do not have the lubrication and the moisture which we find lacking in so much of the food available today, it affects the bowel most adversely.

We know that Grandma always took care of the bowel. She would use sulfur and molasses as one of the old remedies. She would also use enemas to clear a blocked bowel. In days past, people were more familiar with bowel problems and how to care for them. We've gotten away from doing these things today and many people are suffering unnecessary sickness and disease because of it.

This book is offered with the idea that with this knowledge, an individual can learn what is necessary for proper bowel management, and to show the results that can be obtained by just taking care of the bowel properly. No doctor should be without this knowledge; no doctor should practice any system of healing without considering the care of the five elimination channels (skin, lymph, kidneys, lungs, and in particular, taking care of the bowel).

To this end, I give to you the best and most important available knowledge concerning the nonsurgical and drugless restoration of normal bowel function.

CORRECT LIVING HABITS

If we lived correctly, there would be no need to concern ourselves with the bowel. However, most of us are not living right. We don't eat the right foods, we don't get the right exercise, fresh air and sunshine. There are so many things we're not doing right, we can't expect the bowel to function properly. What are the statistics on disease today, and what are doctors doing about it? Virtually all of their attention is directed to treating physical problems and troubles which are products of bad living habits.

Bad living habits are too often picked up from this modern civilization. When I say modern civilization, I am talking about progress, and we all like to think of ourselves as progressive people. But it is obvious that a lot of things we've progressed to are not good for our health, and this is something we must correct. Doctors are not teaching people to live correctly, and they must begin to do this. I believe every doctor should spend half of his time teaching his patients how to live right.

What do our government health departments do? They watch for disease. They are really "disease departments." When an epidemic comes along, they try to take care of it. We give money to organizations and institutions but do they try to find out how to prevent any disease? I see that one organization was given a huge grant to study diet and nutrition and their effects on cancer. So, they are going to start by finding out how alcohol affects cancer. I believe it is reasonable to ask why they aren't conducting research to find out how to help **prevent** cancer. Of course they are going to find that alcohol has a detrimental effect. That is a foregone conclusion. But they're still not going to tell you how to prevent cancer, how to keep from getting it or even how to bring on a remission. So, I believe we must turn around. We must take a new direction in the way we look at health.

AN OUNCE OF EDUCATION IS WORTH A POUND OF TREATMENT

We need to know how to become healthy and how to stay healthy. There are different kinds of people, and we have to reach each of them at their own level of understanding. Some people will pay anything to get well after they are sick. We find as far as health is concerned, you can't pay for it—you earn it. You work for it. So often the average treatments we have today leave the patient void of knowledge, with no change of consciousness. Unless you elevate your mental attitude, your consciousness, you're not taking a better health path.

Too many people with coffee-and-donut lifestyles go see the doctor, get a treatment, then go right back out to that caffeine and sugar habit again. They will be back, you can bet on it! No one in a hospital should ever be allowed to leave until they are given a full day of instruction on how to manage their kitchens at home, how to feed their families and how to prevent recurrence of the trouble that brought them there. Otherwise, they will soon be back in the hospital. You may think I'm a little harsh in this, but every doctor says that one operation leads to another. Do you know why? Because nothing was done to deal with the original cause which led to the first operation.

LET'S OPERATE ON THE PROBLEM INSTEAD OF THE BODY

I ask my patients what operations they've had and almost invariably with everyone, the first is a tonsillectomy. The doctor removes a lymph gland organ and this is one of the organs that eliminates catarrh, phlegm and mucus acids. It is the only part of the lymphatic system that functions to externally throw off what your body can't use. The next operation is the appendix; this is also lymphoid tissue. What's going on here? We don't keep our bodies clean; we don't know how to keep them clean. Cleanliness can begin in many ways but we can't put new wine in old bottles. We can't put clean food into a dirty body and expect good results. We're only going to get partial, perhaps even negligible results. We have to do better than that.

We have been trained to believe that if the bowel isn't functioning correctly we can turn to laxatives. I believe there are more laxatives sold in this country than any other drug with perhaps the exception of aspirin. Cold remedies are very heavy sellers, as are tranquilizers; but you will find laxatives in almost every home. Somebody in each family always seems to be constipated; somebody in the family has bowel trouble. When the children used to get sick, what did grandmother suggest? An enema of course. Grandma and grandpa used sulphur and molasses, and they had many other ways to take care of the bowel. But we find that laxatives are not the solution to bowel problems. We have to go deeper.

7

We must realize that the bowel has the poorest nerve structure of any organ in the body. Having the poorest nerve structure, the bowel can't signal its problems. If you get a little pinprick on the finger you immediately pull away from the pain that causes the distress. But there are no painful distress signals in the bowel because it has such poor nerve reactions and nerve supplies. Where there is a problem in the bowel, and you feel it, you are really in trouble. You must recognize that the average person doesn't take care of the bowel until the very last thing. This was brought home to me especially with the death of the popular movie actor, John Wayne. We find that he first had an operation on the lung. Three months later, he had an operation on the stomach. Another three months and he had an operation on the bowel. We tend to leave the bowel until last.

BACKGROUND EXPERIENCES

Often, parents neglect to teach their children about bowel movements and regularity. I grew up just like Topsy. If I was busy playing, I let the bowel movement go; if it didn't happen today, I'd wait until tomorrow. I had a patient from Brazil who was having a bowel movement every 18 days, and her previous doctor told her that was normal. She experienced menstrual disorders and constant headaches for years and she also had aching shoulders. I knew I didn't have to do anything about these symptoms. Instead, I took care of her bowel. You know, when she started having one bowel movement a day for a month's time, her shoulder pains disappeared and her headaches were gone. After three month's time, she no longer had her old menstrual problems.

I once studied diet and wholistic healing methods with Dr. Glenn J. Sipes in a San Francisco college. One time he received a phone call asking him to see someone in Walnut Creek, California, which is just the other side of Oakland. Because it was an emergency, he agreed to go and asked me to go with him. On arriving, we found a young man about 26 years of age, red as a beet and oozing liquid from his skin. He had extreme pain throughout his entire body and a very high fever. Dr. Sipes tapped the man's bowel with his fingers and asked when he'd had his last bowel movement. The young man said he couldn't remember. Dr. Sipes turned to the mother and asked her to prepare an enema, as the young man needed one right away. She asked what an enema was. Now, here was a mother who didn't even know about enemas! There wasn't a thing in that house to give an enema with, but Dr. Sipes was a man who could always find his way out. He went outside, down to the creek and cut a piece of reed about 2-1/2 feet long. He had the mother fill up a kettle with warm water. He cleaned the pith out of the reed with baling wire, took some of the warm water and blew it into the rectum, causing the man to eliminate. This procedure was repeated for over an hour. In an hour and a half, the man's fever had completely dropped to normal. There was no more redness of the skin and no more pain in his body. The effects of that enema made a powerful impression on me. This is just one experience I've had and I could tell about hundreds more.

Grandmother used enemas to take care of the bowel for the same reason that people in early cultures used herbs. They didn't have any scientific reason for using herbs, but experience showed they worked. They used herb tea for the kidneys because it worked. In Mexico, they use Manzanita tea; in the Causasus, they use Camomile tea. Over the years, the specific uses of herbs have become more or less catalogued so we know what effects they have upon specific organs in the body. Enemas also work. However, I don't think our work in this area is complete.

One of the first things doctors often say is that you can't reabsorb toxic material from the bowel; and I once believed that too. I graduated from college with those ideas, but I found in practice that when we take care of the bowel condition from an enema standpoint, there is a certain amount of water retained in the bowel and immediately after, there is an excess amount of water going through the kidneys. The person urinates a good deal. I began to wonder, was it possible that the water went through the bowel to the kidneys without taking some of the waste material along with it? Years ago, we used to take urinalyses of people and indican was one of the things we always tested for. Indican revealed the toxic material absorbed from some parts of the body, usually from the bowel, and eliminated through the kidneys. Today, indican is not checked in urinalysis. In fact, the bowel isn't considered important enough to take care of. I have seen books in our universities that claim one bowel movement every five days may be considered normal. However, normal in today's world does not necessarily mean healthy.

DETOXIFICATION
The Path to Improved Health

Detoxification is often neglected, overlooked or underestimated in the healing arts, despite the fact that all health professionals realize that a sick body is a toxic body. Toxic acids are normal products of cell catabolism, and we also assimilate varying amounts of toxic material from the air we breathe, the food we eat and other environmental sources. When these can be eliminated from the body, there is no problem. But when toxins are being assimilated or created in the body faster than they can be gotten rid of, or when one or more of the eliminative systems are underactive, trouble lies ahead. I am convinced that toxic accumulations in the body create the necessary preconditions for disease to develop.

DEVELOPING A TOXIC COLON

I believe that when the bowel is underactive, toxic wastes are more likely to be absorbed through the bowel wall and into the bloodstream from which they become deposited in the tissues. If any eliminative system is underactive, more wastes are retained in the body. As toxins accumulate in the tissues, increasing degrees of cell destruction take place. The digestion becomes poor and partially digested material adds to the problem because the body cannot make good tissue out of half-digested nutrients. Proper function is slowed in all body tissues in which toxins have settled. When anyone has reached the degenerative disease stage, it is a sign that toxic settlements have taken the body over. This is the time when we have to consider detoxification—the cleansing of body tissues.

Our bodies can be overwhelmed by toxic accumulations as a consequence of fatigue, poor circulation and improper diet. When we detoxify the body, we must also take care of those things so we aren't simply spinning our wheels. I want to emphasize that an underactive body burdened with toxic wastes does not have the capability of throwing off those toxins. As a body becomes increasingly toxic, proper oxidation cannot take place in the tissues. Without oxygenation, we lack energy and a tired body continues the downward spiral. It can't throw off toxins. Sick people are always tired people.

WORKING TOWARD A HEALTHY BOWEL

Perhaps because of the bowel's central position of importance among the eliminative organs, some health professionals of the past became "bowel minded." We have discovered that it is much better to be "whole body" minded and to start out with a complete tissue detoxification.

A healthy bowel requires sufficient water, good nerve tone, good muscle tone, adequate circulation and the right biochemical nutrients in the right amounts. These, however, are not sufficient to bring health to a dirty, toxic-laden bowel. Cleansing must come first, then tissue rebuilding can take place. This is not an easy task and I don't believe anyone can do a good job in less than a year's time. This estimate is based on the time it has taken to see healing lines coming into dark, chronic bowel areas of the irides after a patient has gone through a cleansing and rejuvenation program.

Our bodies expel a certain amount of toxic materials every day. Medical lab tests have been developed to check whether toxin levels in the blood, urine, feces or mucus are normal. Furthermore, there are tests for the skin, hair and saliva to tell what toxins are being eliminated. By means of these tests, chemical imbalance may be recognized.

THE IMPORTANCE OF PROPER ELIMINATION

Of all the processes essential to good health, we find that proper elimination is certainly one of the most important, and when we consider systems of the body, it is apparent that good bowel management is necessary. I must admit that I did not realize the importance of good bowel care until years of experience in the science of iridology proved to me, beyond the shadow of a doubt, that the condition of the bowel tissue is often the key to the state of health or disease of the individual.

I am convinced and truly believe that our problems begin more in the bowel than any other part of the body. The body depends on a clean bowel. The cleanliness of any tissue, i.e., kidney, stomach, brain, depends upon what is found in the bowel.

ORGANIC VERSUS FUNCTIONAL

There are two conditions in people that I always take care of right away. It is difficult to separate these conditions and yet they represent two ways of treatment.

People are dealing with both physical and mental imbalances and I get to the root of their problem by finding out what they believe in, what is at the bottom of their troubles.

If you believe a lie, then you live a lie. If you believe in happiness, desire happiness and know how to go about attaining happiness, then chances are you are happy. However, the person who holds a vision of themself as diseased, distressed, blue, trapped or unable to get well, has to be reeducated. They have created their own world and trapped themselves in it. Many are victims of percentage diagnoses—"Your chances of getting well are only 30%," and we have to erase this from their mind.

We have an organic condition and a functional condition. When we deal with an organic condition we have to change the tissue, we have to change damaged cell structure, create a new chemical balance, promote better circulation; we have to remove obstructions, pressure and other gravitational effects. These things are strictly physical and we find that the mind alone cannot overcome them very well. I believe that the mind has a tremendous effect on the physical body but that we must feed each aspect its own kind of food. In the organic or physical aspect, we use diet, corrective exercise and tissue cleansing.

We feed the mind or functional aspect of our being with education; teaching people to grow out of their problems, to change their attitude and consciousness. They must learn to walk the higher path in thoughts, words and deeds.

I have changed people's cell structure many times, actually showing them the results with blood tests, but they still hang onto their old attitudes. They want to get well but don't believe they can. This confused state is transferred to every cell in the body. This is why I question people about their mental attitude; we have to see where we are before we know where to go.

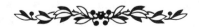

Chapter 2

A BRIEF DISCUSSION OF THE ANATOMY AND PHYSIOLOGY OF THE BOWEL

In order to better familiarize the reader with the scope of this book, the following discussion is provided. Proper bowel management does not require one to be a bowel expert. It is helpful, however, to understand the basics of bowel anatomy and physiology in order to more fully comprehend the message I have to share with you concerning good bowel management.

The bowel responds ideally to the laws of right living as outlined in this book. One must be aware of these laws and persevere to follow them. The rewards in health and freedom from disease are more than worth the effort.

THE SMALL INTESTINE

When food has passed through the stomach by way of the mouth and esophagus, it enters the long, coiled tube called the small intestine. Here is where about 90% of the absorption into the bloodstream of all food constituents takes place. By the time it reaches the small intestine, food from the mouth has been reduced by the action of chewing and digestive juices into a liquid known as "chyme."

Digestion of carbohydrates starts in the mouth with saliva. Further digestion takes place in the stomach. Proteins are broken down into short chains of amino acids (the essential ingredients of protein formation) in the stomach, while further reduction takes place in the small intestine until the molecules can be properly absorbed.

13

When chyme has been thoroughly mixed and broken down by the stomach, the pyloric sphincter muscle valve opens and allows the food to enter into the uppermost portion of the small intestine or duodenum. Here in the duodenum, the first of three portions of the small intestine, the chyme is again thoroughly mixed by the contraction of the muscular walls.

The longitudinal and circular muscles of the intestinal walls are capable of performing three different types of movements, each serving a different purpose. The tube of the small intestine is divided by the circular muscles. These contract, segmenting the food as it passes. Further contraction of the muscles between these segments occurs, making smaller segments, then the first set of muscles relax. This action results in a sloshing motion called *rhythmic segmentation* and takes place 12 to 16 times a minute. As a result of these movements, the chyme is thoroughly mixed with digestive juices. A wave of contraction known as *peristalsis* flows from the duodenum through the *jejunum*, or middle portion of the small intestine, all the way to and through the *ileum*, third and final portion. Peristalsis is the motion caused by the rhythmic coordination of the muscles and propels the chyme through the small intestine. Normal muscular activity of the intestine is not usually felt, although toxin-producing bacteria may cause violent and painful spasms to be felt. Diarrhea and vomiting are both reactions to irritations of the stomach and bowel.

THE DIGESTIVE JUICES

Chyme entering into the duodenum from the stomach is highly acidic. It contains a concentration of hydrochloric acid and enzymes which are required to break down the larger molecules so that absorption becomes more prolific. The small intestine secretions contain bicarbonate, an alkaline substance which causes a neutralization of the stomach acid. Special cells in the intestinal wall secrete these substances and are combined with juices flowing from the gall bladder (bile) and pancreatic juices which flow by way of the pancreatic duct into the duodenum. Bile salts, produced in the liver and stored in the gall bladder, once in the intestine act like a detergent to emulsify the fatty acids and glycerides, making very small particles to be absorbed into the walls of the intestine. By way of hormonal secretions, the small intestine is able to control the digestive processes.

HOW ABSORPTION PROGRESSES

The small intestine is so constructed that nutrient absorption is most efficient. A large inner surface area is provided by the accordion-like folds of the intestinal wall. Lining the wall are finger-like structures called *villi*. They project into the interior of the tube from all directions. The average adult has a small intestinal area of approximately 200 sq. ft. The small molecular particles of the broken down food are able to pass into the cells lining the villi and are taken up by the tiny blood capillaries and eventually find their way into the hepatic portal vein where they are carried to the liver and reduced even further. From the liver, digested food substances are delivered to other cells in the body to support life-giving cellular activities.

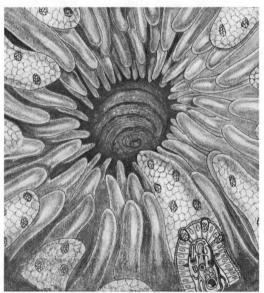

VILLI ARE FINGER-LIKE STRUCTURES THAT LINE THE WALL OF THE SMALL INTESTINE.

Fatty food products do not enter the bloodstream as do other foods. They are taken up from the intestine through ducts in the villi called *lacteals*. Lacteals connect with the lymphatic system whereby these fatty molecules eventually drain into the thoracic duct. The thoracic duct empties into the vena cava in the neck area. This process allows the fats to enter the bloodstream where they pass through the liver for metabolic rearrangement.

In the ileum of the small intestine are found the nodules of lymphoid tissue known as Peyer's patches. These lymph tissues contain scavenger cells or lymphocytes which have a protective function by attacking and destroying unfavorable bacteria that find their way into the intestines.

The small intestine averages 20 to 22 feet in length and is from 1-1/4 to 1-1/2 inches wide throughout this distance. The ileum terminates at the base of the large intestine in the right lower section of the abdomen.

THE LARGE INTESTINE OR COLON

Within 8 to 10 hours of eating, the food has passed through the small intestine and is mostly digested. It then enters the large bowel for the final digestive processes and elimination.

The colon is divided into the following sections: the cecum, ascending colon, transverse colon, descending colon, sigmoid and rectum. Altogether it is approximately 5 feet long and 2-1/2 inches in diameter.

The cecum is a blind pouch whose open end joins the ascending colon as it ascends upward toward the first bend called the hepatic flexure. Here at the cecum is found the ileo-cecal valve, a sphincter muscle which controls the flow of food materials from the small intestines into the large intestine.

Situated at the extreme end of the cecum is the worm-like sac called the appendix. It is about 3 inches long and is often the source of inflammation resulting in a condition known as appendicitis.

The colon, unlike the small bowel, has a mucous lining or membrane which is smooth and void of villi. Surrounding thus mucous layer is a muscular coat consisting of circular internal muscles and longitudinal external muscles as found in the small bowel. The colon is shaped into bulbous pouches called *haustras*. These haustras are made up of muscles which contract to gather the colon up into a puckered appearance and which allow considerable expansion.

The colon terminates in the rectum and anus, the exterior opening. The anus is held closed by the anal sphincter muscle.

The mucus membrane inside the rectum is striated in length-wise segments giving it a fluted appearance. Generally the nerve supply to the colon is sparse and therefore sensory impulses are very weak. Colonic muscular activity is largely unfelt as a result. An exception is found in the rectum where nerve endowment is greater and thus there is the pain associated with hemorrhoids or other rectal disturbances.

HOW THE LARGE INTESTINE FUNCTIONS

Through the ileo-cecal valve, chyme is passed into the cecum from the small intestine. At this stage, the chyme consists of undigested or undigestible food substances, secretions from the liver, pancreas, small bowel and water. In the cecum, the water is mostly removed, reducing the chyme to a semi-solid consistency which is now called feces.

To provide lubrication for the passage of the feces, numerous cells line the walls of the bowel and secrete a mucus substance.

As a result of haustral churning, a constant sloshing effect finishes the digestive process of the chyme. Under mass peristalsis, the feces are pushed toward the rectum and anus where they are eventually eliminated from the body. This movement is caused by the presence of food in the stomach. This activity empties the cecum and makes it ready to receive new chyme from the small intestine.

BACTERIAL ACTION IN THE BOWEL

When the bowel is healthy there is very little bacterial action in the small intestine. The large intestine, however, lilterally swarms with billions of these microscopic organisms.

Bacterial action in the large intestine plays a major role in nutrition and digestion. These friendly bacteria synthesize valuable nutrients by digesting portions of the fecal mass. Among others, vitamin K and portions of the B complex are produced. This aspect of digestion is not completely understood and is undergoing further study. Any remaining proteins are broken down by the bacteria into simpler substances. By products of bacterial activity are numerous, such as indole, skatole, hydrogen sulfide, fatty acids, methane gas and carbon dioxide. Some of these substances are very toxic and odorous, hence the accompanying smell of feces.

The brown color of feces is a result of bile pigments coming from the liver. When feces are not brown, but have a chalky appearance, there is a problem in bile secretion and digestive ability.

When feces reach the rectum they are about 70% water; 30% by weight of the mass represents bacteria while the remainder is made up of food residues, cellulose, undigestible materials and dead cells discarded by the body.

The time it takes for chyme at the cecum to turn into feces and travel to the rectum depends upon the amount of roughage in the food and the water content. Bulkier feces travel faster as they provide substance for the bowel muscle to work upon. Otherwise a soft, fiberless stool becomes very difficult for the colon to move along. The longer it takes, the more water is absorbed, making feces compacted and hard so that it becomes difficult to eliminate them.

Neglecting the urge to eliminate, as well as eating foods low in roughage, will lead to constipation. Laxatives, taken as an aid in elimination, either act to increase the amount of liquid retained in the feces, or act as a lubricant to allow for easy passage. Oftentimes laxatives are compounded to be an irritant or poison and stimulate the muscle walls to cause abnormal contractions to expel the irritating substances. It is very easy to become dependent upon these drugs and thereby permanently destroy normal bowel function.

The expulsion of liquid feces or diarrhea, can be produced by excessive use of laxatives, nervous stress, infection or the presence of toxic substances in the bowel.

Proper bowel management enhances the natural flow and rhythm of the digestive organs providing regular, painless and efficient functioning as described in this chapter.

THE SHAPE OF THE COLON

A healthy, normally functioning bowel is shaped as seen in the illustration on the next page. The cecum is located in the lower right abdomen. From there the bowel rises up into the ascending colon until it reaches the first turn toward the left. This turning point is called the hepatic flexure because of its proximity to the liver. From there the bowel travels across the abdomen beneath the stomach until it reaches the second turn called the splenic flexure. This section of the bowel, the transverse colon, is the only organ within the body that makes a transit from right to left.

In a normal bowel the transverse colon makes a slightly upward grade to the splenic flexure.

From the splenic flexure, the bowel moves down as the descending colon until it reaches the sigmoid colon just above the rectum. Here in the sigmoid is the holding place for feces waiting to be eliminated. The rectum continues from the sigmoid and makes an 's'-like bend into the anus where the anal sphincter muscle is found.

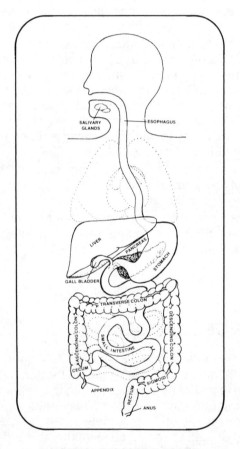

NORMAL DIGESTIVE TRACT

Chapter 3

AUTOINTOXICATION

In the preceding chapter, I discussed the anatomical and physiological functioning of an idealized bowel. Unfortunately, there are many obstacles we must be aware of that interfere with this ideal.

Autointoxication is the result of faulty bowel functioning which produces undesirable consequences in the body and is the root cause of many of today's diseases and illnesses.

If we can make the analogy of the large intestine, or colon being the body's waste disposal or sewer system, we can begin to understand the process more clearly.

Imagine what would be the result of a pump failure in a city's sewer system or what would happen if all the pipes got plugged up with some unmovable material so that the system failed to move waste? It wouldn't take very long before a crisis developed and a huge sanitation problem would threaten health and society.

From open sewers in the past sprang the devastating plagues and diseases that literally destroyed whole cities and populations. When the sewer backs up, we have an immediate health problem potential. Call the plumber!

In addition to the above scenario there is the possibility that the proper functioning of the waste elimination and treatment process can be shut down due to a power failure. The works themselves are O.K. but the energy that feeds all the machinery is shut off or is only partially available. We can liken this to what happens in our bodies when food is nutritionally deficient and fails to give us energy.

All the above conditions are being experienced in our bowels today. Why? The full explanation would fill volumes and volumes. We can distill the main causes for brevity and still get the message however.

Basically, modern civilization, especially the industrialized nations, have the greatest bowel disturbances. We find that native peoples living close to the land and nature do not experience these problems and such diseases as diverticulitis and colitis are virtually unknown.

So what is it that makes these bowel disturbances in our culture? It's hard to point a finger at any one aspect in particular because they are all contributing in varying degrees. Individuals suffer from one aspect more intensely than another due to environmental factors and personal living habits.

In general, the overall major contributing factor is our straying away from a simple, natural lifestyle, wherein all the preconditions for happy, healthy living are found. We find that the further we stray from natural processes and the more we depend upon unnatural and artificial processes our disease and illness increase in frequency and intensity.

In particular, we find that the food situation has contributed most heavily to imbalances in people's bodies today. The way we grow, harvest, process and market our food is at the root of much disharmony in our population.

Economic factors have totally overruled all other considerations in food marketing and distribution. Vital, nourishing, life-giving food simply cannot be had when it is treated as it is today. Unfortunately our foods are hybridized to promote high yields, follow specific climatic conditions, meet harvesting and processing requirements, and have economically advantageous marketing and shelf life characteristics. Nutrient quality, freshness, taste and vitality as it becomes part of the human body is totally neglected. Processed, cooked, dried, roasted, burned, chemicalized, embalmed, preserved foods do not react well in the human body. In fact, they produce very unpleasant things, as you will witness later in this book.

Anyone who is aware of health conditions as they exist today is familiar with the case against the present system of food production. Therefore, let us go on to the other considerations that are responsible for bowel troubles today.

As a result of our poor food conditions, the body is not able to get the proper nutrition. Food grown on poor soil does not have all the vitamins, minerals and enzymes necessary for good health. Our people are growing up with shortages in their nutritional balance. These shortages produce abberations in body chemistry which reflect in disease, illness and unbalanced mental states.

Additionally, processed, devitalized foods are notoriously lacking in fiber and bulk. They tend to be dry, goopy, sticky and pasty. They do not do well in making the transit in the bowel. They have a tendency to stick to the insides like glue and are difficult to move out. A constant diet of this kind of food puts one upon the path to all the things we are going to discuss in this book. Unfortunately this process gets started early in life.

Other factors we should consider in autointoxication are the stresses and tensions put on the members of modern society. When the body is under stress and strain, as is so often encountered today, it needs an extra amount of nutrition to cope with the increased needs caused by this stress. Sadly, the food eaten is so deficient that the body is always in a state of "catching up!" Never getting what is required, a vicious cycle is set up where starvation of vital tissues begins to occur. This situation is in itself stress producing and vitality reducing.

Symptoms such as lack of energy, tiredness, irritability, restlessness, intolerance, quarrelsomeness, fatigue, lack of endurance and increasing frequency of illness are all products of the things I've been discussing.

Now let's combine these conditions and see what happens. First of all, the sewer lines are beginning to get plugged up because of all the glue in the pipes. This causes a backing up of all systems. Waste material is staying around longer than it used to. There hasn't been a reduction in the need to eliminate those materials and therefore the machinery has not had a break, but must instead labor even harder to move the same amount of materials. We find that more electricity is required to do this extra work and all equipment is now operating at a higher wear rate and will require additional maintenance to keep it all going. The possibility of equipment failure has increased due to the overload.

Now imagine a brown out or worse yet, a complete failure in the energy supply. All systems come to a very sticky halt.

When the bowel becomes encrusted with unexpelled fecal material due to poor dietary habits, the absorption of vital nutrients slows down to the degree of encrustation. This is equivalent to a brown out. The energy cycle is short circuited and a downward spiral of tissue integrity ensues.

In addition, the accumulations on the bowel wall become a breeding ground for unhealthy bacterial life forms. They begin to multiply on this putrid, decaying material and the stage is set for serious consequences.

The heavy mucus coating in the colon thickens and becomes a host for putrefaction. The blood capillaries to the colon begin to pick up the toxins, poisons and noxious debris as it seeps through the bowel wall. All tissues and organs of the body are now taking on toxic substances. Here is the beginning of true autointoxication on a physiological level.

By this time, there is little to no existent friendly bacteria in the bowel. The colon has been completely overrun by harmful, toxin-producing virus and bacteria. The sewer is backed up and the power has been turned off. Call the doctor!

It is an indisputable fact that not only illness and old age, but even death are due to the accumulation of waste products of body chemistry and, on the other hand, to the inability of the body to replenish its cellular structures and organs with fresh vital nutrients. Therefore, immunity and freedom from disease can be had and old age and death can be deferred only as long as body wastes are kept at a minimum and fresh, vital material of the first order is supplied for growth and repair of the body.

Colonic cleanliness is of tremendous importance to general health. When the colon becomes polluted with stagnating waste and its tissue becomes damaged by abrasions and infective ulcerations, the end products of poor digestion, lowered metabolism and putrefactive fermentation waste find easy entrance into the blood, lymph and other body fluids.

Beside the morbid conditions already mentioned, one must consider the common and increasing prevalence of diseases of the colon, sigmoid flexure, rectum and anus; diverticulitis, colitis, hemorrhoids, fistulae, fissures and malignancies. These diseases are so serious and are becoming so prevalent that they have created an army of rectal surgeons, colonic irrigators, etc.

COLONIC EXPERIENCE

The benefits of colonic therapy were introduced to me by Dr. George E. Crowle of Los Angeles, California. He believes that the colon is the most important organ of the human body. The sanitary and active conditions of the colon predispose the body to good health.

It was years ago that I went to New York and took up special work with a colonic specialist who had written a book showing that he had put the colon tube completely up the descending colon across the transverse colon, down the ascending colon and had it touching the appendix. I saw this in X-rays and felt as though I would like to study with this man in some of the colonic work he was giving.

He had me do a good deal of this colonic work over a period of a month in his office and I noticed that people who ate certain kinds of food always had a certain kind of a bowel movement. Those who had the natural fiber foods in the bowel always had a well-formed stool and it seemed to pass along fairly well. However, there were very few well or healthy people who came in for these colonics. These people were living on "civilized" foods. One of the things we noticed most was that those people who had a lot of bread were the ones who really had the poorest colon conditions. They were the ones who, when X-rayed, had the most diverticula. We came to the conclusion that anyone taking bread or any of the refined floured products must use a fiber as found from vegetables along with it. To this day, we have followed that program because we saw so many great changes in the elimination of toxic material by colonics when people used vegetable fillings and plenty of them along with their sandwiches.

Today, I believe that no one should eat sandwiches or have any refined carbohydrates of any kind unless they have plenty of fiber material to move it along. Now in many cases I think if we took the natural cereals and natural materials in the very beginning, we wouldn't develop many of these colonic troubles. Of course, we can't tell the average person this, they have to find it out the hard way.

Normal, healthy tissue cannot exist where diverticula exist. We have come to the conclusion that all breadstuffs made of refined flours should be kept out of the body, that means all bread, cakes, pies and pastry. We teach people to use the four cereals that are so neglected in the diet; millet, rye, yellow cornmeal and rice. They must be whole and natural as God gave them to us so that we might have enough roughage to keep our bowel in good tone.

Diverticulosis has increased tremendously and I believe that it is one of the greatest problems for the gastro-intestinal specialist to take care of today.

The following clipping is from the *Daily News Service,* 1981:

CANCER RISK FOR WOMEN

A new study by University of San Francisco medical researchers has revived a turn-of-the-century idea that toxic substances produced in the bowel can have damaging health effects. The study's findings also support recent suggestions of a link between a diet high in fat and low in fiber and an increased risk of developing breast cancer. The study of 1,481 non-nursing women showed that those who are severely constipated tend to have abnormal cells in the fluid extracted from their breasts. Such cells have been found in women with breast cancer and, the researchers suggested, may indicate that the women face an increased risk of developing cancer. The cellular abnormalities occurred five times as often in women who moved their bowels fewer than three times a week than in women who did so more than once a day. Chronic constipation is often the result of a diet high in protein, fat and refined carbo-hydrates (sugars and refined flour) but low in such fibrous foods as whole grains, fruits and vegetables.

In past years, we have taken care of many chronic cases; we have seen remission through natural means, and it has been through cleansing of the bowel to which I attribute my success in these cases. We do not take care of any cancer cases, nor do we treat or counsel cancer patients. We do, however, advise these people to be under the care of a medical doctor. The medical doctors are equipped to take care of these extreme cases; and there are many who are now looking at the wholistic view in caring for the colon.

Chapter 4

CONSTIPATION

This is a subject that everyone talks about, usually experiences, and spends a good deal of money trying to overcome or avoid. Last year, laxative sales were conservatively placed at $350 million. Now that's a lot of constipation! What's going on here?

Over 70 million Americans suffer from bowel problems. The number 2 cause of death in the United States is cancer. Of these, 100,000 give up their lives every year due to cancer of the colon. Here is a quote from the American Cancer Society, *"Evidence in recent years suggests that most bowel cancer is caused by environmental agents. Some scientists believe that a diet high in beef and/or low in fiber is the cause."*

Colon problems such as colitis, ileitis and diverticulitis affect a conservative number of two million people. The medical profession reports that *"Despite decades of research in these diseases, their cause and cure for the most part is still unknown."*

Colostomy is a surgical procedure whereby the intestine is severed from the colon due to that organ's functional breakdown. The colostomized individual is then faced with the lifetime elimination of feces through an opening in their side into an attached pouch. There are 100,000 people who undergo this radical approach each year.

Needless to say, bowel difficulties such as autointoxication and constipation are a growing concern to almost everyone. Out of these two conditions, which are actually symptoms of another problem, come a plethora of evils that are ruinous in their consequences.

Constipation is a clogging up of the large intestine. It occurs in several ways. One of these is by a natural building up of the irritated mucus membrane and bowel wall to such an extent that feces can hardly pass through. One autopsy revealed a colon to be 9 inches in diameter with a passage through it no larger than a pencil! The rest was caked up layer upon layer of encrusted fecal material. This accumulation can have the consistency of truck tire rubber. It's that hard and black. Another autopsy revealed a stagnant colon to weigh in at an incredible 40 pounds! Imagine carrying around all that morbid accumulated waste.

When the bowel is that dirty, it can harbor an amazing variety of very harmful bacteria and parasites. It's interesting to note that worms outrank cancer as man's deadliest enemy on a world-wide basis! It is estimated that 200 million people are infected by these intestinal parasites.

These worms range in size from microscopic single-celled animals to 20-ft-long tapeworms! These parasites kill more people annually than does cancer. One in four peple in the world today is infected by roundworms. The U.S. is not immune to these parasites, as the number of cases has increased in the past few years.

The need for bowel sanitation and cleanliness has been sadly neglected for some time now. Bowel movements every two to three days are considered normal and acceptable. We of the wholistic, nature-cure professions, know better. Our experiences prove beyond a doubt that poor bowel condition is the source for many, many disorders in the body. Recently medical researchers in African countries have had a first-hand opportunity to verify these beliefs.

Both British and South African medical scientists strongly insist that what is usually referred to as "regularity" may be a matter of life and death. Insufficient numbers of bowel movements and too little fiber and bulk in the feces may often explain the existence of gall bladder disorders, heart problems, varicose veins, appendicitis, clotting in deep veins, hiatal hernia, diverticulosis, arthritis and cancer of the colon. This complete turn-around in medical orientation comes from top-notch surgeons and biochemists.

In less than a century, there has occurred an incredible increase in certain diseases which these researchers have attempted to explain by comparing Africans living under tribal conditions and people living under the conditions of Western countries.

Their research indicates that the increase in disease rates in Westerners were caused by changes occurring in the food makeup that reaches the large bowel. In former times, ingested food was much coarser, contained more bulk and indigestible fiber. The processing of foods today makes them mushy, soft, fiberless and bulkless.

These researchers claim that this situation is having a detrimental effect upon the American and British health. In England, Africa and India experiments were conducted to compare eating habits, foods and bowel waste products. These studies indicated that people living under primitive conditions on diets high in indigestible fiber passed from 2-1/2 to 4-1/2 times as much feces as those in the Western countries, and these people were found to be relatively free of most of the diseases studied.

Those studies concluded that diverticulosis appears to be directly related to a high carbohydrate diet such as one containing white flour and sugar.

The long retention of feces is also claimed to be a source of heart disorders, as the removal of fiber from the diet raises serum cholesterol levels and predisposes the body to coronary disease. The accusation is made that the removal of fiber from the diet is also responsible for tumors and cancer due to biochemical changes associated with poor bowel elimination.

Constipation is often referred to by those who have studied the situation as the "modern plague." Indeed, it is the greatest present-day danger to health. Intestinal toxemia and the resulting autointoxication is a direct result of intestinal constipation.

Constipation contributes toward the lowering of body resistance, predisposing it to many acute illnesses and the creation of a great many degenerative and chronic processes. It cripples and kills more people in our country than most any other single morbid condition having to do with deficient function of life. For a lack of the colon to attend to its normal, regular and efficient function almost every human ailment has been attributed.

What disturbs proper intestinal function? It involves a major factor in life—abnormal nutrition. Nutrition is of paramount importance to the general welfare of the body.

Unless the individual educates himself in the art of conscious living, acquires rational habits and lives up to them consistently, nothing but physical and mental catastrophies can be the result.

Intestinal constipation causes cellular constipation. It also increases the workload of the other excretory organs—kidney, skin, liver, lungs and lymph.

The functioning of these organs becomes depleted and overworked. The cellular metabolism becomes sluggish, repair and growth are delayed and the ability to eliminate waste materials is lowered. The cells, instead of being alive and active, become dead and inactive. This process results in a decline in tissue and organ functional ability.

Dr. Alexis Carrell, at the Rockefeller Institute for Medical Research, took small pieces of heart tissue from a chicken embyro to produce one of the most remarkable experiments in medical history. He attempted to demonstrate that under suitable conditions, the living cell could live a very long time, perhaps indefinitely.

The heart tissue was immersed in a nutrient solution from which it obtained its food. Likewise, waste material was secreted into this same solution. Everyday the solution was changed, taking away waste substances and providing fresh nutrients. It is amazing to report that this chicken heart tissue lived for 29 years in this fashion. It died one day when the assistant forgot to change the metabolized polluted fluid! In other words, autointoxication claimed this great masterpiece of experimental scientific investigation.

Said Carrell of this experience, *"The cell is immortal. It is merely the fluid in which it floats which degenerates. Renew this fluid at intervals, give the cell something upon which to feed and, so far as we know, the pulsation of life may go on forever."*

The primary causes of constipation can be summarized as follows: faulty nutrition, ignoring the call to eliminate, lack of physical activity, emotional and mental distress, extrinsic poisons and medications and lack of adequate amounts of water.

Faulty nutrition, as we have already seen, is a major underlying factor in constipation. Processed, devitalized foods low in fiber or bulk are not suitable substances to promote health and well-being. Ignoring the call to eliminate feces or urine contribute greatly to cellular congestion, autointoxication and eliminative organ distress.

The lack of physical exercise makes weak and flaccid muscle tone incapable of holding up under the demands of poor diets and extra eliminative duty. Emotional and mental strain and tension produce unfavorable conditions in the digestive and eliminative organs, causing them to become tense and underactive. These also cause chemical imbalances and abnormal secretions to occur, generally upsetting the whole organism.

Extrinsic poisons, such as tobacco, coffee, alcohol, chocolate and sugar, have unfavorable effects upon digestion and elimination by upsetting gastric secretions and nerve responses. Medications have a very upsetting effect upon these life-giving functions. They cause many afflictions in the bowel. Antibiotics, such as penicillin and sulfa, can completely eliminate the favorable intestinal flora, leaving the opportunity for reinfestation by harmful bacteria and virus. Laxatives are irritating to the bowel and are dangerous if used frequently.

Most people do not drink enough water; they are chronically dehydrated. This causes all body tissues and fluids to become thicker and more viscid. The mucous lining in the colon changes in consistency, failing to provide a slick lubrication for the movement of feces.

Poor living habits contribute a great deal to poor bowel function. Not following a good program denies the body regularity and consistency. It never knows what's coming next and can't depend upon a regular routine. It is always on the defensive. This situation results in a depletion of vital nerve force and undermines the body's ability to set periods of rest and activity.

Today, there are more than 45,000 laxative and cathartic remedies being manufactured and used by Americans alone. Even when used sparingly and in an emergency, these substances should be used with great caution, if at all. The mechanism of elimination is very delicate and easily upset. Once disturbed, it will often require weeks, maybe months, before it becomes regular again.

These substances, in order to evacuate the colon, are essentially poisons and irritants. They contribute nothing to restore normal or natural processes of defecation. The poisoned colon tries to evacuate the offending substance as quickly as possible, and pushes everything out including the compacted feces.

Oftentimes, these harsh poisonous substances are absorbed through the lymph and blood vessels and find their way to all parts of the body. This situation contributes to addiction and overuse of these substances. Dependency upon laxative compounds will in time, permanently destroy the normal ability of the bowel to eliminate naturally on its own accord.

Laxatives tire out the bowel muscle by keeping it constantly working. Without rest, it will soon fail and produce some of the conditions I will discuss in the next chapter.

The only stimulation that the body should have is through exercise. Any time we artificially stimulate the bowel, there is an opposite effect that manifests in which there is a lack of tone in the muscle producing a weakness in that muscle structure.

It is becoming increasingly clear that bowel troubles have a reflex effect upon specific organs in the body. For example, Sir Arbuthnot Lane, who was a surgeon for the King of England, spent many years specializing in bowel problems. He was an expert at removing sections of the bowel and stitching it back together. He taught this work to other doctors and gained an international reputation for his efficiency. During the years of this work, he began to notice a peculiar phenomenon. During the course of recovery from colonic surgery, some of his patients experienced remarkable cures of diseases that had no apparent connection with his surgery. For instance, a young boy who had arthritis for many years was in a wheelchair at the time of surgery. Six months later, this boy had recovered entirely from the disease. Another case involved a woman with a goiter. When a specific section of the bowel was removed in surgery, there ensued a definite remission of the goiter within six months.

These and similar experiences impressed him so much because he saw the relationship between the toxic bowel and the functioning of various organs in the body. After much thought about this relationship, he became very interested in changing the bowel through dietetic methods and spent the last 25 years of his life teaching people how to care for the bowel through nutrition and not surgery.

Sir Lane has said, *"All maladies are due to the lack of certain food principles, such as mineral salts or vitamins, or to the absence of the normal defenses of the body, such as the natural protective flora. When this occurs, toxic bacteria invade the lower alimentary canal, and the poisons thus generated pollute the bloodstream and gradually deteriorate and destroy every tissue, gland and organ of the body."*

I am absolutely sure that what Dr. Lane discovered through his surgical explorations is indeed an accurate description of how the bowel functions in relation to the other organs in the body. We know that every organ and tissue is dependent upon the healthy well-being of every other organ and tissue in order for there to be a total well-being. When one tissue or organ fails, it affects the whole body. If there is faulty functioning in the bowel, this deficiency is passed along to the rest of the body. We could call this the intestinal domino effect.

The frequency or quantity of fecal elimination is not an indication of the lack of constipation in the bowel. I know of cases that had three and four movements a day and yet the bowel was quite encrusted and very constipated. Most people don't know the condition of their bowel. Unfortunately those who are not aware of their bowel function or condition are sometimes the ones who are developing the worst cases of bowel troubles.

I find that constipation is usually going along with those bowels that have diverticulosis. Very few people eat in an organized way, and for this reason, they have loose bowels one day, stiff bowels the next day, a smelly bowel one day, and so on. When regularity is absent in the diet, there is chaos in the bowel. In most cases, simply changing the diet and eating habits will alleviate many bowel problems without surgery.

WHAT GOES IN DOESN'T ALWAYS COME OUT

I am convinced that the bowel holds onto waste materials longer than anyone realizes. When we clean out the bowel and release all this old, rotting material, there will be a lessening of the gas, pain and autointoxication taking place. I believe that this toxic material decaying away in the sigmoid colon is a good place for degenerative diseases to get started.

Starches that haven't been digested properly by the pancreatic secretions are not readily taken up by the body and made into good tissue. These, in turn, can come back to the colon and keep the body from having the proper colonic tone because of a lack of proper chemical development. In addition, drugs can settle in the tissues of the body and it is the colon that catches a good deal of these. By way of the mucus membrane, the colon is used as an eliminative channel. When the membrane does not function properly, these drug deposits accumulate in the bowel indefinitely and can produce a time-bomb effect; irritations, inflammations and ulcerations.

Here again, food is very, very important to recognize because this is the one thing that brings back a chemical reserve and gives the power and chemical structure to have good healthy tissue.

The dietary program that I have developed is probably one of the most important things I can give to you. It has proven itself well in 30 years of sanitarium experience and has helped many people to regain their health. It takes care of the bulk, it takes care of the fiber, it takes care of the natural mucus membrane through proper chemical replacements. This program, coupled with an exercise routine, will produce very good results for those afflicted with bowel disturbances.

THE FUNCTIONING OF THE BOWEL

We have to stop and think that when we eat there is peristaltic action in the bowel which moves the food down to the last part of our elimination system, the large colon. Whenever we have three meals a day and a bowel movement once in five days, we're fifteen meals behind. Normally it takes eighteen hours for food to go through the body and be eliminated. What is required to move it along on time? Good bowel tone gives the power to the intestinal tract to move waste materials properly through the system. If we don't have good bowel tone, we have to have an inciting measure, and one way of doing this is by using laxatives. But we find that 95% of all laxatives are irritating to the bowel, and this is what forces the peristaltic action. It is caused by irritation. Wouldn't it be better to have a bowel that could move along because you have the right power and bowel tone? Wouldn't it be nice to have a bowel wall that has all the potassium and all the right chemical elements to work normally?

We find there are other factors involved here, such as the liver activity. We have to have enough bile coming from the gall bladder and the liver to give the bowel its natural incentive to produce bowel movements. The bowel is dependent upon other organs too. There is also the thyroid gland which is important to the body's metabolism. The thyroid regulates a number of organ functions and keeps them normal by releasing thyroxin into the body. The adrenal glands may be underactive. A person can feel so tired and fatigued that he won't exercise. You have to feel lively to move and get going. An underactive thyroid can bring on low blood pressure and anemia can keep us from a healthy level of physical activity. If the blood is anemic, the body tissue is anemic and cannot do its job. We are tired "all over," so to speak.

CLEANING UP THE PAST

Above all, we now have to make amends for some of the things that happened in the past. I think accumulations in the bowel have to be looked after. The bowel is underactive. It hasn't been fed properly. The bowel itself is probably the most abused organ in the human body. The reason I say this is if you ever go through a cleansing program, you will see things you'll find hard to believe. You don't realize what can come out of the bowel. After just one cleansing treatment, I've seen as much as three gallons of hard toxic material come from a person. How is it possible? I know, for instance, of one woman who said she had five bowel movements a day; but after she passed away, it was found that there was only room enough for a pencil to pass through parts of her bowel. Her bowel was 9 inches across. We found that it had an extreme accumulation of hard toxic material encrusted on the bowel lining.

Constipation is a serious menace to health and vitality as I have discussed with you. The consequences of this common but subtle malady are becoming more and more prevalent in our society. It is a root cause for many troubles in the body. It is also a symptom of a larger picture that many doctors haven't taken into consideration as yet.

The following illustrations show how food moves through the gastrointestinal tract in a 24-hour period and what happens when the bowel doesn't eliminate on time.

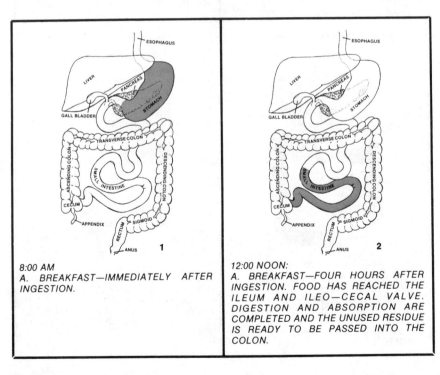

8:00 AM
A. BREAKFAST—IMMEDIATELY AFTER INGESTION.

12:00 NOON:
A. BREAKFAST—FOUR HOURS AFTER INGESTION. FOOD HAS REACHED THE ILEUM AND ILEO—CECAL VALVE. DIGESTION AND ABSORPTION ARE COMPLETED AND THE UNUSED RESIDUE IS READY TO BE PASSED INTO THE COLON.

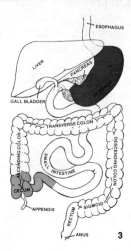

1:00 PM
A. BREAKFAST RESIDUE PASSING THROUGH THE ILEO-CECAL VALVE INTO THE COLON.
B. LUNCH IS NOW IN THE STOMACH.

3

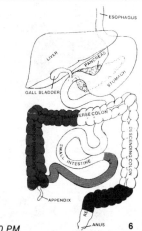

5:00 PM
A. BREAKFAST RESIDUE IN THE COLON.
B. LUNCH RESIDUE IS READY TO ENTER THE COLON.

4

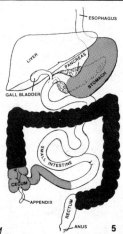

6:00 PM
A. BREAKFAST RESIDUE IS MOSTLY IN DESCENDING COLON.
B. LUNCH RESIDUE PASSING INTO THE COLON—MIXING WITH BREAKFAST RESIDUE.
C. DINNER JUST EATEN AND IN STOMACH.

5

9:00 PM
A. BREAKFAST RESIDUE IS IN SIGMOID COLON, READY TO BE DISCHARGED.
B. LUNCH RESIDUE IN CECUM, ASCENDING AND TRANSVERSE COLON.
C. DINNER RESIDUE IS READY TO ENTER THE COLON.

6

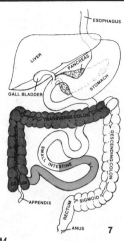

10:00 PM
A. BREAKFAST RESIDUE DISCHARGED
(BOWEL MOVEMENT AT BEDTIME.)
B. LUNCH RESIDUE MOVING THROUGH
COLON.
C. DINNER RESIDUE WAITING TO ENTER
THE COLON.

7

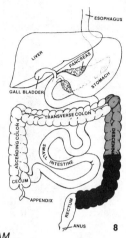

6:00 AM
MORNING OF SECOND DAY
DINNER RESIDUE IN PELVIC COLON
READY TO BE DISCHARGED.

8

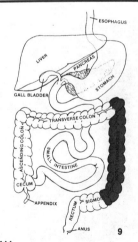

6:30 AM
SECOND DAY
A. HALF HOUR AFTER RISING,
IMMEDIATELY AFTER BOWEL MOVEMENT
B. RESIDUE OF PREVIOUS NIGHT'S
DINNER LEFT IN THE COLON.

9

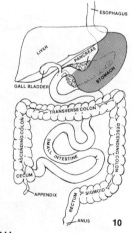

8:00 AM
SECOND DAY
A. BREAKFAST IN STOMACH. BOWELS
HAVE COMPLETELY EVACUATED IN
PREPARATION FOR THE NEW SERIES OF
MEALS.

10

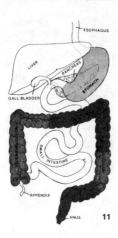

11

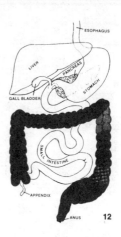

12

DIAGRAM SHOWING CONDITION OF COLON WHEN BOWELS MOVE ONLY ONCE DAILY, CONTAINING RESIDUE OF SIX MEALS.

DIAGRAM SHOWING CONDITION OF COLON IN CHRONIC CONSTIPATION— SHOWING NINE OR MORE MEALS HELD BACK.

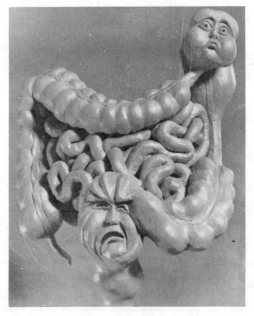

Artist Unknown

Chapter 5

IMBALANCES OF THE LARGE INTESTINE

Structural, functional and metabolic imbalances of the colon are manifested in various forms. We will mention a few of the more common abnormalities of the colon to illustrate the effects of autointoxication and constipation. These are: adhesions, ballooning, colitis, diverticulitis, mucosal dysfunction, spastic bowel, strictures and ulceration.

Adhesions in the colon are caused by inflammations and irritations to the bowel wall. When the mucus membrane breaks down, tissue becomes exposed, open and irritated. The raw surfaces begin to stick together as the result of glue-like substance secreted from the tissue. This is a serious condition and requires delicate treatment to correct.

Ballooning of the colon occurs as a consequence of backed up feces. For various reasons, feces can accumulate and stretch the bowel wall into enormous proportions. This often occurs in the sigmoid colon as the result of a narrowing of the bowel lumen below the ballooning. This narrowing can be caused by adhesions, spasm or colic conditions. When this occurs, constipation can become quite severe and painful and has a damaging effect upon the bowel structure and function.

Colitis is an irritable bowel condition that is highly associated with psychological distress. Few people truly realize the benefits of a calm and peaceful lifestyle. They are often unaware of the mind's ability to sink into the body's functioning ability and upset normal tissue activities. Fear, anger, depression, stress, tension, worries and obsessions can all upset delicate processes in the body, and in particular, those of digestion and elimination. Sometimes what we need is a good cerebral laxative to rid the mind of emotional autointoxication and constipation.

Diverticular disease of the colon is occurring at an ever-increasing rate. It is a serious bowel disturbance leading to many difficulties and must be avoided. When the diet is lacking in bulk or fiber, the colonic muscle must work extremely hard to force feces through the organ. Where there is weakness in muscle fibers a hernia occurs, producing a small pouch or sac-like protrudence in the tissue. It looks like a blister on the side of a tire where the air is forcing its way to the surface through a weak spot in the tire wall.

These sacs, or diverticula, are blind in one end. Therefore feces accumulate within them and hold morbid matter in which a variety of very unfavorable organisms can begin to breed. They become sources of infection, inflammation and degenerative conditions. They are also the host for the production of powerful toxins, adding to an already over-burdened and toxic body. I have seen X-rays of the colon in which there were 142 of these little sacs on one bowel. When these diverticula become inflamed and irritated, we have a case of diverticulitis. Should any one of these festering sacs produce a rupture, then we have a grave situation in which life is threatened by the release of these very poisonous substances into the abdominal cavity of the body where infection can spread quite rapidly.

Mucosal dysfunction occurs when the intestinal mucus lining becomes stagnant and putrefactive. It begins to develop many unfavorable conditions. No longer does it serve the function of facilitating elimination of fecal material. Instead it degenerates in several ways. It can become abcessed, in which case irritations, abrasions, ulcerations and bleeding can occur. Food passage can be very painful.

Mucus can dehydrate and accumulate due to increased viscid consistency. This causes layer upon layer to be built up until extreme constipation occurs. This old material becomes a source of infection and toxic absorption, holding many otherwise excreted products. It also greatly inhibits the absorption of nutrients and water, adding to nutritional crisis.

A **spastic bowel** is often associated with colitis. The point I want to stress is that when bowel muscle or any muscle is overworked, tense and not given an opportunity to rest, it will go into a spasm. Muscle spasm is a chronic tightening of the fibers due to hyperactivity in the nerve impulses controlling muscle action. The symptoms frequently manifest as constipation, alternating with diarrhea. Mental and emotional stresses are high on the list of contributing factors, coupled with chronic toxemia and poor diet.

A **stricture** of the bowel usually occurs after an inflammatory disease such as colitis has damaged the tissue. It is a chronic narrowing of the passageway that often results in a backup of feces that are unable to pass through. The feces accumulate in front of the stricture, causing ballooning, while the segment just past the stricture collapses.

Ulceration of the bowel occurs due to irritations, abrasions, infections and toxic concentrations settling in or on muscle tissue. This results in open sores, bleeding and much pain as is common in hemorrhoids, etc. The sigmoid and rectum are the sites for most of these troubles. Again, autointoxication and constipation are the root causes.

THE FOLLOWING DRAWINGS ILLUSTRATE THE VARIOUS ABNORMAL SHAPES OF THE BOWEL IN COMPARISON TO A NORMAL BOWEL.

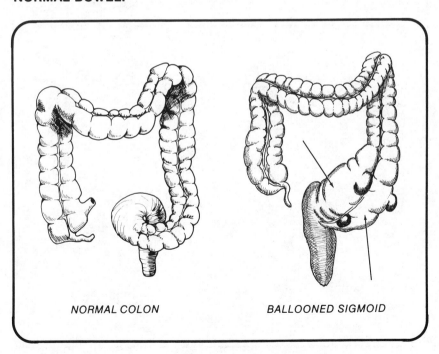

NORMAL COLON   *BALLOONED SIGMOID*

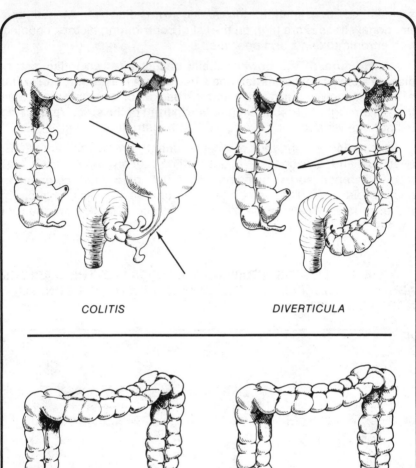

COLITIS

DIVERTICULA

SPASM

STRICTURE

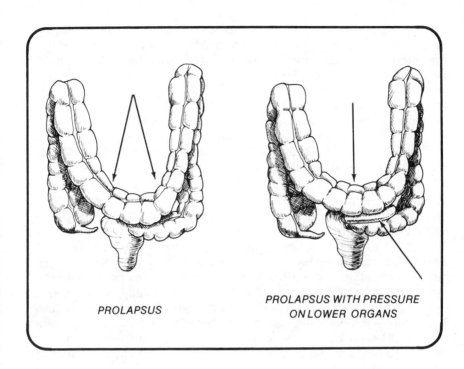

PROLAPSUS

PROLAPSUS WITH PRESSURE
ON LOWER ORGANS

There should be no doubt about the relation between health of the intestinal tract and health in the rest of the body. Intestinal management probably is the most important thing a person can learn in a health-building routine. Some of the most important functions of life take place in the intestines. Through it worn out cells are eliminated and new cell structures have their beginning.

At the Battle Creek Sanitarium I heard Dr. John Harvey Kellogg say he knew of many cases in which operations were prevented by cleansing and revitalizing the bowel. He maintained that 90% of the diseases of civilization are due to improper functioning of the colon. Sir Arbuthnot Lane (M.D.) of London has shown the relation between bowel stasis and disease. He left no doubt as to how seriously he regarded the effects of intestinal intoxication when he said, *"The lower end of the intestine is of the size that requires emptying every six hours, but by habit we retain its contents twenty-four hours. The result is ulcers and cancer."*

Besides these world-renowned exponents of intestinal sanitation, other authorities have given recognition to the belief that cleanliness of the colon is necessary to good health. It is believed that disorders such as appendicitis, infected tonsils, liver and gall-bladder infections, dysfunction of the heart and blood vessels, sinusitis, arthritis and rheumatism, etc., no doubt have their origin in a sluggish colon. There is also an increasing number of morbid conditions in the various parts of the colon, involving the flexures, the rectum and the anus. Consider the amount of surgery and various therapies of hemorrhoids, fistulas, prostate disturbances and malignancies.

While I attended the National College in Chicago many years ago, autopsies were performed on 300 persons. According to the history of these persons, 285 had claimed they were not constipated and had normal movements, and only 15 had admitted they were constipated. The autopsies showed the opposite to be the case, however, and only 15 were found not to have been constipated, while 285 were found to have been constipated. Some of the histories of these 285 persons stated they had had as many as 5 or 6 bowel movements daily, yet autopsies revealed that in some of them the bowels were 12 inches in diameter. The bowel walls were encrusted with material (in one case peanuts) which had been lodged there for a very long time. Thus we see that the average patient coming to a doctor's office does not know whether or not he is constipated.

Some of my patients believe that if they have three bowel movements a day they have diarrhea, and that a couple of movements a week is normal. An example of the latter was a lady patient I had who assured me that she had normal movements; that her bowels moved regularly, every Tuesday and Friday morning. Most people have not been properly educated in their childhood to realize the importance of adequate daily elimination and to heed nature's call to evacuate the rectum. This indifference to the natural urge to evacuate the bowels may be the beginning of constipation.

Doctor John Harvey Kellogg, who gave us so much of his philosophy and practical experience, lived to the age of 91. Since he did more work in connection with intestinal sanitation than anyone in this country, his advice should be worth listening to. It was his opinion that we should eliminate the residue of each meal 15 to 18 hours after eating it. Babies, savages, birds and animals evacuate a short time after each meal.

Observe from the following statistics published by the Register General of England that no group has contributed more to the death rate from intestinal diseases than doctors.

"Comparative Mortality from Diseases of the Digestive System."

Physicians, surgeons	50
Inn-keepers	45
Barristers, solicitors	44
Seamen	43
Clergymen, priests, ministers	34
Butchers	30
Car men, carriers	28
Farmers	25
Gardeners	22
Railway guards, porters	20
Agricultural labourers	19
Average among all workers	28

As shown by the above statistics, the death rate of doctors is 31 points higher than that of agricultural laborers, and 22 points higher than that of the average death rate of all workers who die of diseases of the digestive system.

Is there a way that these troubles can be avoided? Yes there is. Early detection will help in many cases, but the real remedy is found in changing the diet and ways of living.

In the meantime, there is only one way that we can do this and that is by making sure that everyone has an X-ray to see if these conditions actually exist. We believe that practically everyone has bowel troubles in the civilized world today due in part to the way we are eating. We can't usually sense these things because the nerve supply to the bowel is so poor that we don't know we have a serious problem until we have pain. Any time there is pain in the bowel, it is a serious condition.

Whenever there is gas, and it cannot be taken care of through the ordinary food routine or through ordinary treatments, then we know it is very serious indeed. I believe that long before any of these symptoms appear in the body there are preconditions in the bowel and we should be able to see how to take care of these things before symptoms appear.

If a person is going to check up on the presence of diverticula possibly the best way is through the barium enema X-ray. This is one of the finest ways of doing it. There should always be two X-rays; one when the bowel is full of the barium meal and one taken after it is emptied. Years ago, I was very astounded when I took a picture of the bowel. We could see that there was some of the barium meal in a little pouch or diverticulum. A week later, another X-ray was taken of the same patient for a gall bladder scan. Upon examination of the negative we were able to see the barium meal still settled in various diverticula throughout the colon. If barium meal can stay there for a week, what happens when food stays there? There is no food that should stay in the colon constantly and over a period of a week's time.

We find through the work in iridology that most diverticula have settled in the sigmoid colon. We feel that this is the logical place due to the fact that the patient hasn't answered nature's call in the past. Bowel accumulations from not only one, two but from ten even fifteen meals have backed up because many people are that much behind in getting rid of the toxic wastes that develop from the food they eat. We find that many patients are having only one bowel movement a week; some two bowel movements a week. I had a patient who had a bowel movement every eighteen days and was still consuming three meals a day.

The driest part of any stool is always in the sigmoid colon. Because of this condition, the sigmoid colon has to withstand the greatest amount of pressure in trying to get rid of this dry stool. With the toilet designed the way it is, it becomes even a greater strain on the sigmoid than on any other part of the intestinal tract. It is here that we find the driest material working the greatest hardship on the mucosa of the bowel wall itself.

Further we find that the kinds of foods that man is eating today are excessive in meats and the putrefactive materials—the heavy additives cause greater irritation. In addition, there are the spices, especially black pepper, which are considered quite an irritant to the colon and to the liver. Many of the coal tar additives develop into drug accumulations as a result of ingesting into our bodies the various nostrums that are so readily taken from the drugstore without prescription. We find that the sigmoid colon is the greatest place in the bowel for these things to settle. Further, we do not bring children up to realize that bowel movements are the most important thing to take care of in the body. We get busy; we let things slide—we put things aside; we "cannot take care of it now."

The refining of carbohydrates has removed the lecithin, oils and vitamin E from these foods. These act as a lubrication when present. The lubrication is not sufficient in refined foods to keep the feces moving for proper elimination.

I believe that diverticulosis is a civilized disease. It is a disease that has come about by our wrong living habits.

It isn't a matter of not having enough fiber one or two days, it is a matter of not having it over a period of many years that can produce this diverticulitis. We find that fast living—not chewing our foods properly; going to the quick-snack shops and eating foods that lack bran (the hull or outside coating), and taking the skins from potatoes, apples, pears, peaches and vegetables deprives the bowel of adequate bulk and fiber. We are eliminating the fiber that we would naturally have to eat and which could well be the basis of giving the bowel wall all the exercise that would be necessary to keep it from forming a diverticulum.

People have gone from the smooth diet of pancakes, pasta and many of the other soft foods that we have today to those of extreme roughage and have caused many disturbances. We believe that by taking our time and slowly changing over from the soft diet to a more rough diet, we can eventually diminish and remove the effects of the diverticula that have been built over many years of wrong eating habits.

FLATULENCE OR BOWEL GASES

Certain chemical processes in the colon produce various gases as by-products of normal bowel function. Some are odorless like carbon dioxide, while others are very odorous such as hydrogen sulfide.

Bowel gases are of no consequence in a healthy colon. This isn't true in a diseased colon, however. Excessive gas is an indication of bowel disturbances and can be very serious in its consequences. For example, when there is a bowel stricture or obstruction due to constipation, the gaseous products may become trapped, not being able to exit the anus. Extreme pressure may develop, causing pain, swelling and other symptoms to appear.

Gas production does not always come from a normal metabolic process. In fact most gaseous wastes are the result of abnormal conditions in the bowel. They are the products of inferior processes at work in the body. Specifically, they are the result of putrefactive fermentations.

When undigested proteins find their way into the colon, they provide nourishment for unfavorable bacterial growths. These undesirable bacteria and virus are responsible for the breaking down of organic compounds by way of a putrefactive process. This process is undesirable specifically due to the fact that these organisms produce toxic, poisonous, disease-producing (morbid) by-products as a result of their metabolic functions. The waste materials they produce are injurious to body tissues. These organisms were not intended to inhabit the human body. Those that are beneficial and indeed necessary for good health cannot live in an environment which is dirty, toxic and constipated.

When there are pockets, diverticula and ballooning in the bowel, there is non-moving waste accumulating in the colon. These conditions are ripe for putrefactive fermentation to occur and result in considerable flatulence, discomfort and seepage of toxins into the body.

A healthy colon produces little to no flatulence.

Taking care of gases in the bowel has been one of the most difficult problems to handle from a nutritional standpoint. When we start changing the diet and go into the natural fibered foods that nature has given us, and leave off any man-handling, we find that we have *more* of a gas condition. It is like the stirring up of a dirty basement and as we brush it clean, there is a lot of dust that has formed. The one unusual thing I observed in taking care of people with a lot of gas is that they could go to town and eat the worst diet possible and they would be free of gas. You could put them on coffee and donuts and nothing but that for 2 or 3 days and they report no gas whatsoever. And, when we put them on a natural fiber diet, as prescribed in our diet advice, then we have gas to contend with. However, they began to say they were passing off the gas easier—their stools became softer; they did not have to force the bowel movement; they did not have to cause pressure; the feces moved easier through the bowel and they no longer were having problems with constipation. However, the gas still persisted, but it seemed to get less and less and, over a period of three months, we found that it came down to a minimal amount.

Once a bowel has diverticula, it will never become totally free of gas. There are very few people who can say they have no gas whatsoever. To get the gas out completely is almost an impossibility in this day and age because we cannot live the way of life necessary to accomplish that task, but I do think it can come down to a minimum and will cause no disturbance—no distress.

THE EFFECT OF GRAVITY ON THE BOWEL

An important thing to realize is that we have pressure, both mechanical and chemical, to take care of as far as the bowel is concerned. On the chemical side, we have the effects of the acidophilus bacteria, acids and putrefactions. On the mechanical side, we have peristaltic action and the ever-present downward pull of gravity. Gravity, we must realize, brings on more problems than most people can possibly imagine.

Do you remember the historic landings of American astronauts on the moon? Were you watching television when it showed them on the moon's surface, easily jumping 10-12 feet high? When they walked, you could see them bounce with each step. They looked like they were bouncing on a trampoline, because gravity on the moon is much less than here on earth. Gravity on earth is very harsh on our bodies.

When we walk or stand, our body is pulled down toward the earth. We have to live with this constant tugging on our vital organs. We find that the intervertebral disks are being pressed down. I'm sure we would have few disk problems if everyone lived on the moon, because there wouldn't be enough pressure from its gravity to cause disk problems. On earth we have gravity problems, especially when we are tired.

I have said before that tiredness is the beginning of every disease; that is when gravity has its greatest effect on the body. When we are tired, we begin to lose muscle tone, so we find that internal organs are more easily pulled downward. When gravity takes its effect, our shoulders begin to droop; we can have scoliosis or we can develop curvature of the spine. The softest tissue in the body is the transverse colon, and it is the only tissue in the body that goes completely from the right side to the left side of the body. If it was made of bone, it would stay in position; but since the colon is made of very soft tissue, a prolapsus or dropped transverse colon can happen as a result of gravitational pull. There is a new disease coming; it's called gravitosis. The symptoms are as follows.

PROLAPSUS OF THE TRANSVERSE COLON

When we have prolapsus, all the organs above the transverse colon are going to fall as well and those below it will suffer the effects of pressure. When the transverse colon comes down, for example, bladder pressure develops. The uterus can develop flexions and retroflexions and could double over the bowel causing constipation. We sometimes find that there is pressure on the fallopian tubes or the ovaries. Many times the egg from the ovary cannot pass into the uterus properly and this can cause sterility. Still further, we find that women have more cysts on the ovaries than on any other organ in the body. There are more hysterectomies given to women than any other operation; and I believe it is because a good deal of pressure is against the tubes, pressure which does not allow proper circulation of blood or the removal of toxic material. But women are not the only ones subject to pressure-caused troubles; a man with a prolapsus experiences prostate gland pressure. The urethra, through which urine flows from the bladder, passes through the center of the prostate gland. When there is pressure on the prostate gland, urination is difficult. There will be retention of urine, which is one of the liquids we can absorb back into the body. This can mark the beginning of arthritis and joint troubles, especially as we grow older. So we find we can have prostate gland and bladder troubles, uterine and ovarian disturbances, all because of prolapsus caused by gravity.

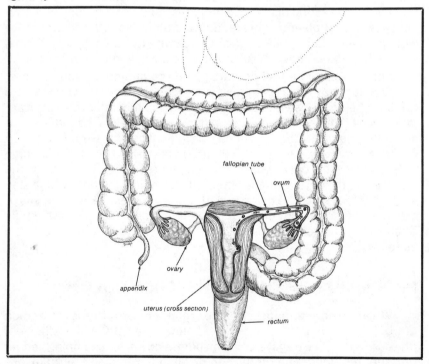

NORMAL COLON AND UTERUS. NOTE NORMAL POSITION OF STOMACH.

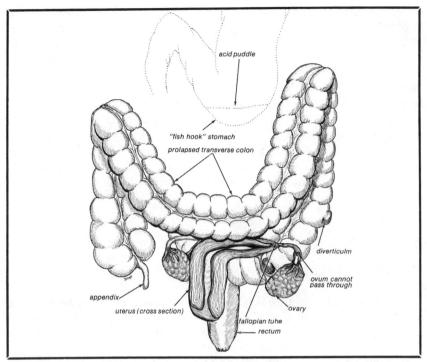

PROLAPSED COLON WITH PRESSURE ON UTERUS. NOTE THAT OVUM CANNOT TRANSIT FALLOPIAN TUBE DUE TO PRESSURE. UTERUS CANNOT PASS MENSTRUAL DISCHARGE EFFICIENTLY. PROLAPSUS OF TRANSVERSE COLON ALLOWS STOMACH TO DROP—RESULTING IN "FISH-HOOK" STOMACH.

Many doctors and gastro-intestinal specialists are making their living treating hemorrhoids and other anal, rectal and bowel problems caused mainly by pressure from the transverse colon and various organs involved while we are eliminating at the toilet. I think the toilet is the most abominable device ever invented in our civilization. We find that the Indians never had any rectal troubles; they had no hemorrhoid troubles whatsoever. Why? They squatted to defecate. If you go to France, Italy or South America, you will find that the toilet is often a hole in the floor and you have to squat. This is the normal eliminating position, the one in which all of our internal organs are held in the proper position. When this position is habitually used for elimination, no veins will protrude from the rectum.

Now to add to the problem, we may have gas or we may have a hard stool. There is pressure against the rectum whenever we have hard fecal material or excessive gas. These problems are aggravated by fatigue and by the gravitational pull. It is well that you know this so you can learn to overcome these things. To overcome the problem of gravity when and if you must sit on the toilet, one thing to remember is to keep your hands over your head. You'll find when you push down, the force is really against the rectal tissues and the rectal areas, so to overcome this keep your hands above your head. That's the way it should be done anyway, if you're going to use the regular toilet seat. In fact, in our sanitarium we had a little rope above and off to the side of the toilet to hold when there was a bowel movement, which kept the hands above the head.

IRIDOLOGY AND THE BOWEL

In looking at the bowel from the standpoint of iridology, the first thing we have found is always a black area in that portion of the iris corresponding to the bowel. The condition of the transverse colon (which comes across the top of the bowel) is indicated by signs near the top of the iris at from 10 o'clock to about 12 o'clock, within what is called the autonomic nerve wreath. We start down the descending colon, represented in the iris from 12 to 5 o'clock, then the sigmoid colon from 5 to 7 o'clock, until we come to the rectal area about 7 o'clock. This is only one side of the body. I don't want to give a lesson in iridology but I would like to take you on a little learning trip because the iris has much to teach us about the condition of the bowel.

In the iris of the eye, various conditions show up as black areas, which I call "bowel pockets," where the autonomic wreath makes a definite break. I have found that the black area represents underactivity, an inherent weakness and a toxic material settlement. Over the years, I went after these three things in my work with patients. I found that an inherent weakness in the bowel quickly leads to problems in bowel function unless the body has all the power and energy it needs to work with. When the body is tired, an inherent weakness in the bowel leads to hypoactivity. So, I had to take care of the energies of my patients. I had to take care of enervation. I had to get rid of tiredness. I had to help patients get rid of what I call "vitality wasters." Every sick person is fatigued and rundown. They are burned out. They want to lie down.

51

Some of them don't even have the energy to walk. All they want to do is to go bed. They don't have enough energy or spirit to really do things, and I found that while taking care of these people, having them rest and change their diets, I began to see certain healing signs come into those black areas in the irides. These correlations between bowel condition and the appearance of the iris were confirmed repeatedly over the years.

THE FOLLOWING DIAGRAMS ILLUSTRATE BOWEL SIGNS AND OTHER IRIS SIGNS AS THEY RELATE TO VARIOUS CONDITIONS IN THE BODY.

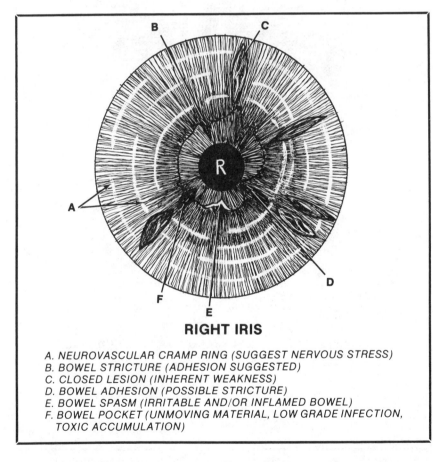

RIGHT IRIS

A. NEUROVASCULAR CRAMP RING (SUGGEST NERVOUS STRESS)
B. BOWEL STRICTURE (ADHESION SUGGESTED)
C. CLOSED LESION (INHERENT WEAKNESS)
D. BOWEL ADHESION (POSSIBLE STRICTURE)
E. BOWEL SPASM (IRRITABLE AND/OR INFLAMED BOWEL)
F. BOWEL POCKET (UNMOVING MATERIAL, LOW GRADE INFECTION, TOXIC ACCUMULATION)

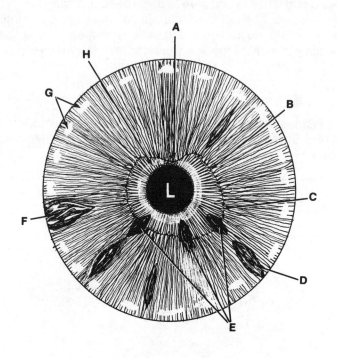

LEFT IRIS

A. PROLAPSUS OF THE TRANSVERSE COLON
B. AUTONOMIC NERVE WREATH
C. BALLOONED BOWEL
D. CLOSED LESION — NOTE PROXIMITY TO BOWEL POCKETS AT 'E'
E. BOWEL POCKETS (DIVERTICULA SUGGESTED)
F. OPEN LESION (INHERENT WEAKNESS)
G. LYMPHATIC ROSARY (LYMPHATIC TISSUE ENLARGEMENT SUGGESTED)
H. ACID STOMACH RING

THE FOLLOWING PICTURES ILLUSTRATE BOWEL ABNORMALITIES AS SEEN IN X-RAY PHOTOGRAPHS.

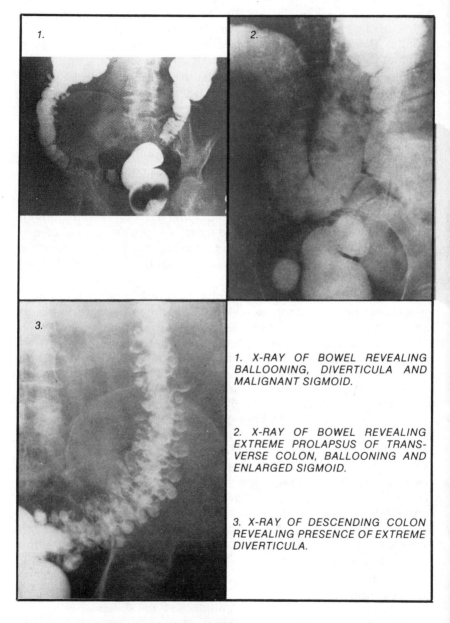

1. X-RAY OF BOWEL REVEALING BALLOONING, DIVERTICULA AND MALIGNANT SIGMOID.

2. X-RAY OF BOWEL REVEALING EXTREME PROLAPSUS OF TRANS-VERSE COLON, BALLOONING AND ENLARGED SIGMOID.

3. X-RAY OF DESCENDING COLON REVEALING PRESENCE OF EXTREME DIVERTICULA.

There is much cynicism among medical doctors over the value of iridology, but I believe this will change. It takes three months to demonstrate healing signs in the eye and the average medical doctor seems to be unwilling to take the time for this kind of systematic follow-up. I can prove what I have presented here, but it does take three months. The average doctor wants to see it right now; he makes one test and that's it. If it isn't there in a week, it doesn't exist.

Iridology deals with tissue changes. When we examine the iris, we are "reading" tissue condition. We do not directly read toxic material settlements in the bowel. When we examine the iris, we are reading the bowel wall. When the healing signs appear, they are called calcium luteum lines. Improvement in the bowel wall takes care of toxic materials in the body; it moves them along a little quicker. We may quicken elimination of the acids by using foods containing potassium and sodium. We find that magnesium relaxes the bowel for those who have tension. Of course, we often resort to using milk of magnesia for this, but we can also use the magnesium which is found in our foods, of which yellow cornmeal contains the most. Magnesium is also found in all vegetables. Using the proper foods to bring about physical changes is slower than drug therapy; it is the natural way. We find no "undesirable side effects" here.

When I first began seeing these changes come about in the irides of my patients' eyes, I actually didn't know I was doing anything unusual. I was simply putting my patients on a right-living regime. But I then started to have X-rays taken, because I wanted to confirm what I suspected was going on. I spent time at the Battle Creek Sanitarium and began to see how the X-rays verified what I was finding through iridology. When my iris reading indicated a bowel pocket at 3 o'clock, I found on the X-ray that there was a diverticulum in the bowel. I found there was a ballooned condition where the toxic materials were not being eliminated as they should. At that time, I studied with Dr. John Harvey Kellogg, who was a master of taking care of the bowel. He wrote on colon hygiene and also did a great deal of work with diet. One thing I learned was that we have "friendly" bacteria in the bowel. These friendly bacteria keep the bowel clean from putrefaction and fermentation which produce excess gas and bad odors. Dr. Kellogg taught that the bowel should be about 85% acidophilus bacteria and 15% bacillus coli, or those which produce gas. This, he stated was the right bacterial balance for a healthy bowel.

I wanted to test my patients for this bacteria balance, so I sent fecal samples from 500 of my patients to a medical laboratory to find out about the relative amounts of acidophilus, bacillus coli and acid-fast bacteria. I wanted to know the effect of the pH (acidity/alkalinity value) and to find out all I could about the intestinal flora. The lab results averaged 85% bacillus coli or detrimental bacteria as compared to 15% of the acidophilus. It was just the opposite of what is should be to be healthy! These were the results for 500 of the patients who had come to my office. Obviously, the bowel of the average patient was not what is should be.

I have taken care of bowel problems through colonics. I have recommended colonics frequently to my patients, but you see, this alone doesn't bring healing lines into the eyes, because healing signs come when there is a new chemical balance in the tissue. I deal in tissue, and when I see various bowel conditions indicated from the eyes, I can't tell you that the problem is always diverticula. It could be diverticula and I would say 9 times out of 10 it is, because X-rays I have examined have demonstrated it as such.

It is so important to mention that through iridology I have found reflex conditions from problems in the bowel. There is a definite relation between certain organ conditions and the bowel conditions as indicated in the eye. For instance, I examined a lady who had torticollis (a wry neck) and when I told her I would have to adjust her neck, she refused because she'd had several adjustments to her neck and it only seemed to become worse each time. She just couldn't stand to have anybody touch it again. Well, I'm a chiropractor and I'm supposed to do adjustments. I was just starting in iridology but I had to do something, so I checked her eyes and found a black pocket. When I asked if she had ever had bowel trouble, she said she'd had it for years ever since her neck trouble began. Lately, the bowel problem had become worse. I prescribed an enema right away. She had three enemas and in one hour's time while I was still there, she obtained complete relief from the stiff neck problem. I walked out of there and I hadn't touched her neck. I only took care of the bowel. This was quite an experience and I will never forget it.

Another patient came to see me some months later who had a large abscess on his neck, and in looking into the iris of his eye, I saw a large black hole with the most beautiful healing signs coming into it. I know you cannot have healing signs unless there is a change in diet. It is very necessary to talk about food. He said he had been driving behind a citrus truck which overturned and spilled oranges all over the road. When he stopped to help, the truck driver told him to pick up as many as he wanted, so he filled the trunk of his car and drank orange juice for 45 days. This certainly was an extreme elimination diet, but he couldn't get rid of the accumulated toxic material in his body fast enough through normal elimination because he wasn't doing enough in taking care of the bowel. The overload of toxic material being eliminated produced the abscess on his neck.

INHERENT WEAKNESSES

Inherent weaknesses are areas of the body where toxic materials finally accumulate. It is in these organs that infection develops. We can have an infection in the lung, we can have abcessed teeth, we can have these problems in various parts of the body, and invariably, these infections come originally from the bowel.

I have found a striking correlation in my iridology studies over the last 45 years, confirming that there is a definite relationship between conditions in sections of the bowel and conditions in other specific parts of the body. When a patient complains of a breast condition, there is a certain place in the bowel that I suspect harbors a low-grade infection which is affecting the breast area; or, other areas of the body may have problems that can be traced to the bowel.

Why separately treat any organ in the body if we find that the source of the problem is in the bowel? Look again to John Wayne. Is it possible that he should have been treated in the bowel area before the stomach and lung? I wonder also about the famous comedian, Jack Benny, who had a perfect examination just two months before he died of cancer. Could his death have been prevented?

In one instance, a boy came to me with left leg problems. He had been treated for three years with massage, mechanical and chemical treatments. Examining the iris of his eye, I found a section of the sigmoid colon, the last part of the colon before it goes to the rectal area, that was quite black. Since we cannot identify a disease from the iris, I refused to treat him until he had an X-ray. He had not had an X-ray until that time. It was discovered that he had cancer of the sigmoid colon and this boy died six months later. I believe this tumor was causing the reflex conditions in his leg, but he had been treated only for the leg problem. I've had many experiences in which black areas in patients' irides showed specific troubles in various organs in the body, and I've been able to verify these in thousands of cases.

I have seen many good results from caring for the bowel. I haven't confirmed complete relief coming only from colonics. I've seen relief, but if you don't change the diet, I don't believe colonics are worth anything. If you don't take care of your marriage problems or financial disturbances, I believe you can create more acids, more mucus problems and more disturbances with distressed bowels, colitis and ulcers. With all the technical treatments available today, I believe we have to consider a complete cleansing that's physical, mental and spiritual.

At the Battle Creek Sanitarium, they showed that you have to have a sufficient amount of the acidophilus bacteria, the friendly bacteria, as compared to the bacillus coli or the gas-producing bacteria. There are certain foods that produce and help to develop friendly bacteria and there are certain foods that break down friendly bacteria. Meat can break down friendly bacteria when you consume too much, especially when you have a static bowel or a lazy colon. We find that coffee destroys the friendly bacteria in the bowel more readily than anything. Chocolate also breaks down the friendly bacteria, as do over-cooked foods. We should be working toward cleansing the body through better nutrition, more exercise, by changing our life habits and go in a direction that will be good for our whole body.

Someone will ask, I'm sure, why we use coffee enemas if coffee breaks down the acidophilus? If one is in need of a coffee enema, chances are that the acidophilus is already gone, and the benefits obtained by its stimulation of elimination are very worthwhile. We reestablish the flora with implants after the cleansing.

This takes courage, determination, perseverance and faith in the ultimate, unseen outcome. Yet, by following the right path, by looking to nature as our model, we realize that our choice has the best potential for health and happiness.

It calls for a commitment to give up the old familiar, easy, toxic habits and take up the new, unknown, seemingly difficult unfamiliar ones. Changing habits is the hardest task in the world to accomplish. It's as if we were made of quick-setting jelly, fresh and pliable right out of the jar, but soon to turn hard and brittle.

There is a fear factor involved in giving up an old habit. Even though it's bad for us to keep it there is still the comfortable feeling in knowing it. A bird in the hand is worth two in the bush—but if the bird in the hand is a vulture, it may end up eating you some day.

Don't commit intellectual suicide by closing yourself off to alternative possibilities, for after all, if what you know and do now is killing you, then you are suffering from a lack of knowledge and wisdom and the saving answer to your problem is to be found in the new, unfamiliar territories.

Alvin Toffler in *Future Shock* aptly states that man's current and future task for survival is in his ability to adopt new ideas and habits very quickly, in fact, much more quickly than he has ever managed in the past. Is he up to it? Can he let go of the life-snuffing old ways quickly enough to recover from past and present mistakes in order to grab hold of a correct and viable alternative? No one knows. We are in the midst of finding out.

We should not accept anything that is not in balance with nature into our bodies. We cannot improve upon God's perfect order. It is suicide to try. It serves no good purpose and is destructive in all ways. Whole, natural and raw is the absolute perfection that our bodies require and respond to best. Anything else is a cheat and a robber.

Processed, white sugar, for example, literally leaches out of the body certain substances. It requires energy and metabolic substances pulled from the body's bank account of nutrients to deal with it once ingested. In return, the sugar gives an incredible nothing. That's correct, nothing! In fact, it takes more to get rid of it than it gives and is therefore a thief of potent proportions.

CHEMICAL IMBALANCES

When the body begins to lose its balance in any sector, there is a reverberation throughout the whole organism that feels that vibration of imbalance. Illness and disease are states of disharmony in the body.

One of the subtlest forms of imbalance in the body that I know of is a chemical or nutritional imbalance. It's like not seeing the forest for the trees. We live in it, on it, and by it, immersed in it to the point of nonrecognition, especially if it is a chronic condition as it so often is.

Chemical deficiencies and imbalances are at the root of many ills. We can even say that the imbalances extend into the atomic level and even on into the electromagnetic levels of cellular function.

Why is radiation so dangerous? Because of the disturbance it causes in the tissues on an atomic level. The chemical processes are upset and influenced disharmoniously. The natural, God-given, peaceful, beneficial order is broken.

When we have toxic substances in the colon seeping into body tissues, it's like having a time-release poison in your bowel. It works slowly, imperceptibly wearing down the vitality, resistance and health of body tissues and organs. It's sort of like having our own personal chemical dump that we carry around with us all the time. It's always working as long as the toxins are present, serving out its lethal microdoses.

Never before has man been in such a toxic, poisonous environment. The air, water, food, soil, clothing and everything he touches has potential or real toxic substances that eventually find their way into the body.

People are more toxic today than ever in known history. The levels of it and the extent of it are becoming a nightmare as illness walks the land.

The need to detoxify and cleanse the body has *never* been greater than right now. Nearly all the patients I see have a toxicity problem that has to be cared for first.

Restoring balance, peace and harmony is the physician's job. That is the task he has chosen to do. It cannot be done effectively or lastingly in a body that is breaking down due to an accumulation of toxic materials in the body; i.e., autointoxication.

When the bowel fails, the whole body goes into a nutritional crisis. Metabolic shock waves flow to every cell and tissue.

It's often said that you are what you eat. I say that you are what you absorb. You can eat the finest foods and still starve to death if the digestive and absorptive processes are not functioning properly.

When we cleanse and remove the toxic debris, feed the body good, healthy, vital foods and stop poisoning ourselves, the body will respond with healing and reversal of disease processes.

We find that the bowel wall needs sodium, which neutralizes acid. The average person produces much acid in the body and this draws sodium out of the body, through the tissues of the bowel and stomach. Furthermore, we know that potassium is very necessary, because it is a muscle element. The average person does not realize that potassium neutralizes acids. To neutralize acids in the body, potassium is taken from the bowel wall. I believe that the bowel wall is the most maltreated tissue of the body, functioning in a constant state of semi-starvation for chemicals which are consumed in day-to-day living. The most important elements found in the bowel wall must be kept in constant supply or we will suffer the consequences.

In addition to the blood and chemical elements, we must discuss some of the foods we put into the body. Bran is very popular now in this country. We should have been using bran all along. Why did we give it up? We have thought a great deal about "junk foods," and we talk a lot about them. We talk about school lunches; we talk about hospital snacks that are available while you're trying to get well. We find that so many of the sweetening materials in drinks today rob the body of the vital health producing elements that are stored in the bowel.

CARE FOR THE MUCOUS LINING

The bowel wall has a mucous lining, and this mucous lining throws off toxic material, acids and catarrh. In order to get rid of the catarrh, the mucous lining has to come off along with it. In most cases, it does not. We find that the mucous lining is not moving out the accumulations as it should, and in fact, it clings to the bowel wall itself. We find that we have to take care of that mucous lining.

The bowel wall may also have an inherent weakness. When I say that I've never found a patient who didn't have an inherent weakness in the bowel itself, I'm not saying that the whole bowel has an inherent weakness, but only sections of it. This shows up as slow and underactive functional ability. If we have food that does not go through our system as fast as it should, we find that it will go still slower and be even more underactive in moving through an inherently weak section of the bowel.

CHEMICAL STRUCTURE

A healthy bowel contains sodium, potassium and magnesium for proper functioning. These three chemical elements are lacking in our civilized foods more than anything else. Sodium is a chemical element that neutralizes acids and it is found in the lymphatic system. It is required in tissue that is pliable, active and movable; i.e., joints, ligaments and tendons.

Potassium is the great alkalizer in the body and found more in the muscle structure than anywhere else. Potassium is found in our bitter vegetables which so few people ever eat anymore. Sodium and potassium are found more in salad vegetables than anywhere else. Salads have been left out more and more in our food intake in recent years and the soft foods taken in their place have increased. Could this occurrence be partially responsible for much of our diverticular and bowel problems today?

We find that magnesium is the relaxer in the bowel; it is also the element most necessary to have good bowel movements. Milk of Magnesia, which is probably one of the most prominent of all drugs being used today, is a good peristaltic stimulator; however, we are using a drug that only gives symptomatic relief.

I do not believe that the magnesium used in its drug form is particularly favorable to remaking and rebuilding the bowel structure. It is the magnesium in our foods that can do the greatest amount of good. Magnesium is found a good deal in salad vegetables. It is found heaviest and most abundantly in yellow corn. Cornmeal is one of the foods that has been milled and refined so much that it no longer has the roughage from the kernel that makes it one of the great laxatives and one of the great bowel toners we can take into the body.

In spite of this shortcoming, I believe that everyone should have yellow cornmeal cereal at least two mornings every week.

As we work with eliminating the encrusted mucous lining, we must also consider nourishing the new cells below it.

We use flaxseed and psyllium seed as a lubricant and bulk. These seeds, along with sunflower seeds and other seed oils, contain vitamin F, which is used to rebuild the mucous lining, especially in the bowel. Thus, we are getting triple benefit from these substances.

MENTAL ATTITUDE

There is a mental side to physical health. The mind can cause tension. We know that it can cause contraction in the bowel wall. We might say that colitis begins in the head. Inflammation of the bowel can be caused by nerves and stress. Many people have much better bowel movements when free of emotional pains and aches and when free from money worries. Good companionship, relaxation and music can be conducive to good bowel movements.

What I'm pointing out is simply that the bowel has to be taken care of through the wholistic healing art, rather than by some drug, adjustment, reflex therapy treatment or even by taking care of the diet. Each of these will bring some improvement, but we must realize that the bowel will not function right until we know how to live properly. There is a way of right living, and it isn't just food or diet. We find that it is important to get along with people, because the problem isn't always **what** is wrong with you; it may be **who** is wrong with you.

I do not wish to give the impression that I have become one-sided in my emphasis upon the importance of a healthy, clean intestinal tract, but evidence has been coming to me for a long time which indicates that people do not realize that constipation is at the root of most of our diseases today. I feel that people are not regarding poor health as seriously as they should. They place their health problems secondary to all their other problems—financial, domestic, real and invented—while the health of an individual or a nation should at all times have first place on the list of duties and responsibilities. Without health there is little that one can truly enjoy.

The road to health is the one that begins with an understanding and commitment to cleanse and detoxify the body, to restore balance, peace and harmony. We must be willing to rise above selfish habits, realizing that the path of cleansing has implications for the intellect, emotions and spirit. We need to accept our personal responsibility on this path.

Chapter 6

INTESTINAL FLORA AND BOWEL GARDENING

Too few people in our culture experience the benefits of proper bowel function. Too few people live in a manner that enables them to maintain the natural balance of the body. Therefore, if we are going to live unnaturally, it would be wise to learn what is necessary to counteract some of the maladies that we create in our personal environment.

Sometimes I wonder if a person can ever be truly happy or healthy while living in a city where natural processes are so disturbed, and often absent altogether. Are we trying to keep people well against all odds?

The medical arts today spend much time and money patching up the effects of an environment that is actually toxic and hazardous to health. Most of today's doctors are treating people for ailments that are direct results of "civilized" living. These "environmental ailments" are reaching epidemic proportions, and rather than eliminate the cause of the disturbance, it is a case of keeping people going while they continue to addictively tear themselves down.

True, lasting and abiding health is the result of conscious discipline in cleanliness of body, mind and spirit. All else is a compromise.

When the body becomes polluted with toxic substances, those forces that maintain health and vitality diminish in proportion to the extent of the invasion. As they diminish, the morbid (disease producing) substances flourish. Such is the case with intestinal flora.

Intestinal flora are those micro organisms which live in the bowels of man. There is a great variety of these microscopic life forms and they play a very important role in health and disease.

Where health and vitality are found, we invariably find the friendly and beneficial microbes. Where there is decay and disease we find the organisms that perform this function. There is no aspect of earthly life in which these life forms do not have an important role to play. They are everywhere; we literally live in an ocean of them. They work unceasingly to bring about the transformations that they are designed to produce.

To a large extent the flora in the bowel determines the state of health in an individual. The large bowel is in fact a mobile compost heap, constantly giving up finished compost and taking on new materials for treatment.

As everyone knows, a compost heap is a very special thing. Here is where the waste products of living things, both animal and vegetable, are collected for the purpose of promoting a process of decay and breakdown. When the process is completed, we have the finest beginnings for new life to get started. Out of the old and dead, comes the new and alive.

What is at the interface of this paradoxical phenomenon? Bacterial and micro life forms. They are the recyclers, the transformers. They are nature's labor force, accomplishing some of the most complex chemical reactions known to man. We are constantly trying to copy or somehow utilize the processes they are capable of producing.

Some of the deadliest substances in existence are produced as metabolites of these bacteria. All life upon the planet is affected by their presence.

It has been determined that the colon contains not only 400 to 500 varieties of bacteria, fungi, yeast and virus, but that the populations vary from the center of the colon to those living in the mucous lining; from those inhabiting the right side to those that inhabit the left side of the bowel.

Research has found evidence which indicates that the mucus secreted by the intestine very much determines the kind of bacteria that will grow there. In addition, it has been found that it takes more than a year on the average for a new diet to produce any noticeable change in the flora.

Of those things that greatly alter the bacterial life in the colon, drugs are the most powerful.

In particular are the "broad spectrum" antibiotics. It has been found that antibiotic-treated animals have higher blood cholesterol levels.

Those bacteria which help control cholesterol levels are killed off by the drug. These drugs can also cause inflammation of the intestinal wall. Antibiotics will, as a rule, wreak havoc in the intestinal ecology, and should, if possible, be avoided. In addition, there is an immunity reaction that can occur in which the body develops an inability to utilize the drug, therefore putting the beneficial qualities of it out of reach. Overuse develops this syndrome and makes it ineffective in many cases. Penicillin is one in particular that has seen much abuse and in a time of great need, may prove to be powerless in many people.

WHAT CONSTITUTES POOR INTESTINAL FLORA?

Those things which man loathes most, morbid substances, are the same things provided by bacteria that can and do live in man's intestines. I believe the preponderance of unfriendly bacteria in the average American bowel would reach as high as 85%.

Bacillus coli is considered to be the king of the court, providing the most offensive reactions. There are many others. The opportunity to have such a guest is facilitated today because of the dietary habits and quality of foods we are using.

Flatulence is produced largely by these organisms. Their chemical reactions are hazardous to the well-being of the body. These substances are very toxic. Very small amounts of specific compounds can produce bizarre reactions in the body. They cause disharmony in the body, chasing away the life force. They are hazardous to living organisms, constantly occupied in breaking down tissue and reorganizing it.

The average bowel provides an ideal environment in which these organisms flourish. We have unwittingly provided the breeding ground on a mass scale by the lifestyles we live. Basically, Western man through the use of technology has so adultered his food that it no longer promotes the friendly bacteria, rather it nourishes the destructive bacteria.

Bacillus coli prefer an alkaline environment, with protein for breakfast, lunch and dinner. A dark, warm, moist place rounds out their habitat. Undigested protein reaching the colon is perfect food for these bacteria; they thrive on it. We literally feed them and promote their growth this way. Meat in particular provides this medium. When these conditions are met, and it doesn't take long, we are opening the doors for guests of this sort. They can invite most chronic diseases man is aware of. They are not good boarders. They are always taking more than their share and never pay the rent. They are not easily evicted and oftentimes claim the whole house from its landlord.

How can we best avoid these things? Ideally, we should never get into this situation. Bowel hygiene should be taught at an early age by our parents. It should be common knowledge and our government should be made responsible to see to it that it is part of our educational system. Those practices and processes that contribute to degeneration should be avoided, and those who promote such abuses should be reeducated.

Until such an ideal is realized, we must deal with the problem the best way we are able according to our individual beliefs and morality.

We can begin with a total cleansing of body tissues in as much as the art has progressed.

Releasing the grip of toxic substances in the body is no small task. It takes work and perseverance, a willingness to release the old and embrace the new.

Fasting, elimination diets, enemas, colonics, herbs, massage and all the healing arts are in one way or another trying to do the same thing; release from the body some undesirable substance whether it be a negative attitude, spastic muscle or lead accumulation, those things that cause disharmony in the body.

Bowel cleansing is an essential element in any lasting healing program. The toxic waste must be removed as quickly as possible to halt the downward spiral of failing health.

This is best done by (1) removing accumulated fecal material from the bowel; (2) changing the diet from a toxin-producing process to that of an elimination and cleansing diet; (3) fasting; (4) colonic flushing with enemas or colonic irrigations; and (5) cleansing the mind of old habit patterns. This sounds like a big order to handle, but it shouldn't be at all. Going slowly but surely in the right direction is the main successful ingredient. Don't try to do it all at once. Too much change too fast causes disorientation, a disease known as future shock.

It is best accomplished by surrounding yourself with the right people—people who are knowledgeable about these things and have your best interest at heart.

A disagreeable, uncooperating spouse or parent can be a major roadblock to success. It may require changes in your life that go very deep. Many people give up rather than change, and ride out the consequences of their decision the rest of their lives.

Once the toxic environment in the colon has been purged by cleansing and elimination; the diet corrected; and all efforts directed toward balance, the body will begin to respond by deeper cleansing of all tissues. The elimination reactions brought on by cleansing, proper and vital nourishment and a change in attitude are a vital part of the rejuvenation process.

As this process proceeds, the house is being prepared to receive new guests. Slowly, but surely, the bowel flora will change with constant encouragement. The once alkaline, high protein, putrefactive environment will change over into one of cleanliness and sweetness, where peace and harmony reign.

IN SEARCH OF THE LACTOBACILLUS ACIDOPHILUS

Throughout known history, man has been enjoying the benefits of a particular food renowned for its health qualities. It provides, in part, substance to every good aspect of human health. It gives endurance, vitality, strength, long life and cheerfulness. It responds wonderfully in the digestive system, promoting every good quality of a healthy bowel.

This food is soured milk. Bacterial action in the milk produces a chemical reaction which digests the milk substances, and makes them an ideal food for the human body. The bacteria that cause this reaction to occur are known as lactobacillus, acidophilus, bulgaricus, brevius and saliveria. There are others, but these are the most widely known.

These are the friendly bacteria to the human body. They provide many wonderful qualities for the organism. First of all, where they live abundantly, the other kind do not or cannot. The acidophilus gets its name from the fact that it loves an acid environment. An acid bowel environment is one's best defense against unfriendly bacteria.

When we provide a favorable environment for the acidophilus, we are at the same time wiping out the breeding environment for the bacillus coli.

So, the process in many respects is aimed at reestablishing the naturally occurring lactobacillus acidophilus. This bowel condition is the one from which man's greatest health can be obtained. Maintaining this condition puts one upon the path to healthy and vital living.

When I say that we want to reestablish the naturally occurring acidophilus, I mean that the acidophilus is normally established at birth. Within the mother's milk is a substance known as colostrum. This substance produces a baby's first peristaltic action in the bowel. Being the first nourishment ingested into the system, mother's milk produces an acid environment in the colon. This occurs due to the lactose or milk sugar that reaches the colon.

When a mother breast feeds her baby, she gives it the best possible start in life and health.

The first bacteria to enter the child's digestive tract will establish itself within a matter of hours from birth. It is now that a very critical decision has been made that will influence the growth of the individual for its life's duration.

If the colon is found to be acid, promoted by mother's milk, then the acidophilus will take root and flourish. If the colon is found to be alkaline or neutral the chances of bacillus coli to flourish are encouraged.

The lactose of mother's milk has the unique quality of being slowly metabolized by the body. It reaches the colon still intact and provides nourishment for the acidophilus bacteria.

Formulas other than mother's milk deprive the colon of this food and therefore set the stage for coli inhabitation—the beginning of disease. Ask around and compare illnesses with those who have been breast fed and those who have not.

Even if one is fortunate to have come in with this natural blessing, it is no guarantee that it will stay that way. Defoliation can occur quite easily. Poor dietary habits in particular cause this destruction of the acidophilus environment. Also, antibiotics will cause great damage.

Lactobacillus bacteria has a symbiotic relationship with the human body. It is a good boarder and always pays the rent in advance, doing more than its share.

When we properly care for the bowel, we are automatically providing a welcome home for those favorable life-giving bacteria that are essential to good health.

Among other things, they provide very valuable nutritional metabolites for the body to use in rebuilding and maintaining health. Examples are portions of the vitamin B complex, enzymes and essential amino acids, the increased and more efficient absorption of calcium, phosphorus and magnesium. They are responsible for the synthesis of certain vitamins. They maintain an antibacillus coli environment. They contribute to good health in many ways we are not scientifically aware of yet.

THE VALUE OF LACTIC ACID

Milk, when first secreted from the udder of a healthy cow or other lactating animal, is sterile, but it becomes   invaded by bacteria almost immediately.

Milk is a good medium for breeding bacteria of all kinds, good and bad. Any changes which occur in the milk after it is secreted are the result of bacterial action converting nutrients into other substances. If bacteria could be prevented from contaminating the milk drawn from the udder, it would remain sweet indefinitely; but this is an impossibility.

John Harvey Kellogg performed an amazing experiment demonstrating this fact. He immersed a one-pound piece of raw meat, slightly tainted, in buttermilk. The milk was changed at regular intervals. The meat remained perfectly free of decomposition for some 20 years!

This demonstrates the efficiency of an acid medium in inhibiting decay producing, putrefactive bacteria.

Soured milk is also called turned, fermented, curdled and clabbered milk. The Bulgarians and Turks called it yogurt; the Russian calls it Kefir.

Among the essential goods of some Nomadic people is a lump of casein milk curds, wrapped up to prevent its drying. This lump of casein is put into the milk bag containing the freshly drawn milk and allowed to remain there until the milk sours. Then the curd ball, rejuvenated in the process, is returned to its wrapping. Using this process, the Nomad knows his soured milk will not rot nor putrefy. In this condition, the milk retains its food value until it is used up.

In more recent years, since the studies of Metchnikoff, fermented milk has been in great demand and widely used. It has been prescribed for better health in general and for a wide range of ailments, particularly those arising from intestinal and metabolic disturbances.

"Metchnikoff is really the father of modern-time fermented milk. He made it popular and as the head of the Pasteur Institute in Paris stimulated a great deal of scientific study about the remedial value of fermented milk. He was an indefatigable worker on the subject of longevity. His experiments for attainment of better health and longer life attracted world-wide attention. He maintained that stasis and putrefaction of the bowel shortens life and causes diseases, early senility and premature death for which he recommended fermented milk best neutralizer and antidote.

"He deduced this from the fact that the Bulgarians, Turks, Arabs, Jews and others who are addicted to the use of fermented milk as the English are to the afternoon tea, produce more centenarians than any other nationality, Bulgarians showing 1,500 centenarians out of every million of population. In America, only nine out of every million reach that age. No doubt the fact that these people use a great deal of fermented milk, and because it contains the very valuable lactic acid and the changed proteins, can be considered as a factor in their longevity. But, lest we forget, how about their simple fare, simple mode of living, the outdoor life they lead! Are these not just as important, perhaps more so, as factors in longevity than just fermented milk?

"Metchnikoff inferred that their longevity was due solely to the fermented milk. He obtained a microbe which he called Bacillus Bulgaricus from the casein ball the Bulgarians used to induce souring in freshly drawn milk of their herd, and found it would indeed induce souring of milk, and very rapidly. He tried to implant this Bulgarian bacillus in the intestinal tract of man, and thereby induce lactic acid formation, thus eventually to crowd out the malignant microbe that may be causing putrefaction, but the experiment was not successful. The Bulgarian bacillus is a milk parasite. Many bacteria produce lactic acid, but relatively few grow well in the alimentary canal.

"Time, observation and experimentation have proven that the bacillus bulgaricus is not viable, which means that when ingested, it does not thrive in the gastro-intestinal tract, but it is digested and destroyed in the stomach and small intestine and does not reach the large intestine. It does not get into the colon where it is most needed.

71

The bacillus bulgaricus after being ingested, does not appear in the feces when examined.

"Lactobacillus Bulgaricus preparations have been omitted because they contain an organism foreign to the intestinal tract of man and incapable of being implanted in the human intestine. The lactobacillus acidophilus preparations have been retained because this organism is capable of implantation, growth and lactic acid-production in the intestine of man.

"The presence of any bacillus acidi lactici in the feces is the only real proof of their value as definite remedial agents in colonic disturbances, especially in constipation. Out of the more than one hundred species of bacillus acidi lactici, including the bacillus yogurt, streptococcus lacticus, thermophilus, lactobacillus adondolyticus, Boas Oppler bacillus, lactobacillus lopersici, etc., none thrive or can be implanted in the large intestine, other than the lactobacillus acidophilus.

"Rahe made a critical investigation of the implantation of L. bulgaricus. His work tends to show that although L. bulgaricus milk is ingested, it disappears very soon after ingestion has stopped. This investigator also points out a very significant fact—that the difference between L. bulgaricus and certain acid-forming bacteria, which are known to occur normally in the intestines, is so slight that they can be distinguished only with difficulty. He suggests that the belief on the part of some investigators that L. bulgaricus becomes established in the intestines was caused by their inability to distinguish between these two types. The only bacillus acidi lactici that can thrive and can be implanted into the adult large intestine is the lactobacillus acidophilus.

"Lactobacillus acidophilus belongs to the aciduric lactobacillus group which is widely distributed in nature. This group of bacteria contains many varieties of related organisms. Lactobacillus acidophilus and lactobacillus bifidus are found in the gastro-intestinal tract of man and animals. Lactobacillus bulgaricus usually occurs in the intestinal contents of cattle. It is frequently present in dairy products, contaminated with fecal material from cows.

"The lactobacillus bifidus predominates in the infant colon. It keeps the child from developing many infant diseases, and makes him also immune to many diseases, as long as he is fed on breast milk, for then the colon is normally acid in reaction. But as the child grows older and the change of diet takes place, proteins are increased at the expense of carbohydrates and sugar—milk sugar. As a result, unfriendly bacteria begin to enter the colon, such as the bacillus coli, the B. Welchii, B. putreficus, streptococci fecalis, etc. Putrefaction and fermentation now are in order. Thus toxic material—indol, skatol, phenol, ammonia, phenylsulphate, ptomaine, pyrrhol, cadaverin, isoamylamine, ethylamine, idroxyl-phynel, and other poisons—swarm in the large intestine.

"Within the past 50 years methods have been developed for changing the nature of the germs that live in the intestines. Metchnikoff's original idea that the bacillus bulgaricus was the normal inhabitant and that its presence was synonymous with long life has been changed to emphasis on another germ called the B. acidophilus.

"As already hinted, with the exception of the lactobacillus acidophilus, all other species of bacillus acidi lactici are not viable; that is, when imbibed, when taken by mouth, they are digested and destroyed in the stomach and small intestine, and, therefore, do not reach the colon or, if they do, their number is negligible. L. Acidophilus is a normal inhabitant of the intestinal tract and under the influence of the ingestion of lactose or dextrin can be made to predominate the intestinal flora. The ingestion of L. Acidophilus milk with or without added lactose brings about the transformation of the intestinal flora more quickly and is generally conceded to be the most logical and practical method of bringing about the preponderace of L. Acidophilus type of bacteria in the intestines. By administering L. Acidophilus milk implantation the proliferation of the organisms in the intestinal tract are more rapidly accomplished for then there is direct implantation of large numbers of viable organisms. The lactose of milk induces the multiplication of the desired type of bacteria.

"It is necessary that large quantities of very active cultures should be taken, and special measures must be adopted to supply to the B.

73

acidophilus, when in the colon, the carboyhydrates which it requires for efficient growth.

"The growth in the large intestine of lactobacillus acidophilus depends solely on starch and sugar, but more so on milk sugar. In order to change the intestinal flora, it is best to adopt the following rules.

"For fifteen days, about eight ounces to sixteen ounces of culture of lactobacillus acidophilus, in which three large tablespoonsful of lactose is dissolved, should be taken daily thirty minutes before breakfast; and for the same length of time, three large tablespoonsful of lactose should be dissolved in any kind of fruit juices, milk, soups, broth or water, and taken daily thirty minutes before supper. After this, four ounces to eight ounces of lactobacillus acidophilus culture, in which three tablespoonsful of lactose have been dissolved, should be taken every morning for fifteen more days. The lactose, however, should be taken as before. After this, the quantity of the culture of the lactobacillus acidophilus can be reduced to four ounces every day for fifteen more days. For the remainder of the time, the ingestion of the culture of the lactobacillus acidophilus, two ounces every day, may be sufficient to keep the required amount of lactobacillus acidophilus present in the large intestinal tract. One must remember that the amount of the daily requirement of lactose, should continue to be about three tablespoonsful, morning and evening, as the daily requirement.

"As to the length of time that the lactobacillus acidophilus culture (together with the lactose) should be taken in order for one to gain the desired results depends on the severity of the condition that is being treated. However, a period ranging from four to six months may be necessary. A period of about three months of rest may be taken and then the procedure, if necessary, may be repeated. It is possible that the taking of the lactobacillus acidophilus culture and the rest periods may have to go on for some time.

"When is the intestinal flora changed? The intestinal flora is changed when the stools are soft, frequent (three times a day), and free from putrid or rancid odor. Examination by a bacteriologist should give positive 80 and negative 20, which means 80% of the acid formers and 20% of other bacteria. In a bad flora, the percentage will be the reverse, 20-80. Of course, a change from 20-80 or worse to 40-60 or 50-50, is a decided improvement, but this should not be considered at all satisfactory. Old troubles may still continue, perhaps somewhat modified. But when the change reaches 75-25, marked improvement will be evident, and the more complete the change of flora, the more decided will be the change for the better in the patient's symptoms.

"The advantages of regularly using lactobacillus acidophilus together with the lactose mixture are obvious. Through not a cure-all, yet one would be temped to say that it should be used not only when diseases have already made their inroad, but more so as a preventive of disease.

"A few more suggestions about the lactobacillus acidophilus therapy. The culture, to be effective, must contain at least 200,000,000 lactobacillus acidophilus per cubic centimeter. Although clinicians experience has been that lactobacillus acidophilus therapy has to be taken in large doses to be effective, there have been cases in which daily doses even as small as four ounces has proved satisfactory when it was mixed with a like amount of lactose.

"In about 75-80% of non-complicated constipation, lactobacillus acidophilus therapy has given uniform good results.

"The lactobacillus acidophilus culture should be used within or before the expiration date marked on the bottle." *

---

*"The Intestinal Flora in Constipation" by N. A. Ferri, Sr., M.D., Chicago, IL.

INTESTINAL FLORA

Current research into intestinal flora of the human bowel has revealed some new and valuable information for the health-seeking individual. (See Bibliography for further reading.)

Dr. Paul Gyorgy of the Institute of Nutrition Academy of Medical Sciences of the USSR (discoverer of vitamin B-6), has determined that the main component of the normal intestinal flora of man is lactobacillus bifidus. Bifidus bacterium readily establishes itself in the colon of newborns when fed mother's milk. It is bifidus that is found in the nipple of lactating mothers. Very encouraging research in both the USSR and Germany have demonstrated the rejuvenating qualities of this bacteria when it is well established in the colon.

The only commercially-available form of **lactobacillus bifidus** that I am aware of comes under the brand name of **Eugalan Topfer Forte,** and can be found in your health food stores. If **not locally available,** address your inquiry for this product and information to: **Bio-Nutritional Products** (see **Bibliography**).

A program using this bacteria following the former instructions should bring encouraging results to those who suffer from a lack of proper intestinal flora.

Everyone should take a good replenishment of acidophilus culture, which can be purchased at any health food store. I recommend taking this culture regardless if you have been on the colema treatments or not. However, it is strongly recommended to be taken after the colema treatments.

Chapter 7

NATURAL METHODS AND TECHNIQUES FOR BOWEL IMPROVEMENT

A WHOLISTIC APPROACH

There are many detoxifying agents which may be useful under various circumstances, but we need to approach detoxification from a "whole body" perspective. We need to do more than just take care of the bowel or liver. We must have the right chemical balance for the body. It is not sufficient to use a drug to provide a chemical stimulus to "drive" the body to work right. Rather, we must repair, rebuild and regenerate the body as we go along. Proper breathing is important to get oxygen to the organs and tissues of the body. Exercise is good to get the blood and lymph circulating but too much exercise in a toxic-laden body is only stirring up muddy waters.

Lymph drainage is important. Drainage can be increased through the use of protomorphogens or through the use of herbal substances such as blue violet tea. Stimulating increased lymph drainage, however, is not sufficient to carry off toxins that may be pouring into the lymphatic system via a stagnant bowel holding five or six meals before elimination takes place or from a bowel pocket holding a mass of putrid material which is being reabsorbed into the body. We dilute the God-given power of our body when the bowel does not eliminate eighteen hours after each meal.

BACKGROUND STUDIES—MY PREVIOUS WORK

Rather than restating work that I have written in the past it would be beneficial for the reader to study four of my previous books. These give a good background for the work that is presented here.

For instance, if you really want to know how to take care of colitis, you should know about the liquefied salads. They allow bulk to get into the bowel in a liquefied form that is more easily digestible. Unfortunately people do not chew well enough—some have dentures or missing teeth that make mastication difficult—others are just lazy. Liquefied salads are a way to get the food reduced to an easily-assimilable size. The book *Blending Magic* tells how to prepare delicious foods that retain their full enzyme and nutrient values.

Doctor/Patient Handbook describes the reversal process and the ways of taking care of the colon through that process.

Nature Has A Remedy is a book that covers the ways of building the body wholistically through the use of herbs, sunshine, fresh air, water and the right mental attitude. When we take care of the "whole" body with these natural, God-given remedies, every tissue and system is revitalized.

A New Lifestyle for Health and Happiness gives a complete program for aligning the body, mind and spirit to the good life. Complete with menus, diet control and comprehensive, self-check analysis.

In an effective bowel management program, you will need to drink at least three glasses of liquid before breakfast every morning. Keep in mind that cold water will stop at the stomach, but warm or hot water will go directly to the bowel. If you want to go on an elimination program, you can use the Velco 77 or 79 bulk and clay water. Follow directions, and use it three times a day with meals over a period of 30 days. You can add more juice to your diet during that time, and you should always take juice after the bulk and clay water. If it is possible, get into some extra bowel elimination through enemas, perhaps using clay water and coffee instead of plain water. This is a kind of elimination program you can use while still working at your regular job.

There are other ways to help the bowel, and I have mentioned taking care of the mental attitudes as well as conditions in the body. Both are very important.

THE BENEFITS OF ALFALFA TABLETS

The second thing I emphasize in the bowel management program is the taking of four alfalfa tablets with each meal. As far as I am concerned, this is almost a panacea. Some health professionals may think I'm going a bit overboard, but I want to tell you that alfalfa tablets provide an excellent natural fiber bulk, and by stimulating the bowel to work against the fiber, we begin to compensate for inherent weakness, by building better tone. Juice is not suitable for this purpose because pulp or bulk is necessary. Some will say that you should take the alfalfa tablets along with additional chlorophyll; I don't find this necessary, because there is chlorophyll in the alfalfa tablets as well. Chlorophyll is a great deodorizer, a great builder, a great acid neutralizer and one of the greatest foods for feeding acidophilus bacteria. I use alfalfa tablets mainly to get into the bowel pockets. I am sure this approach is right, because since beginning to use it, I have observed more healing signs associated with the bowel from my iridology analyses than anything I have ever used. Of course, I'm kicking a lazy dog; I'm kicking a lazy colon.

Now, we may encounter a few minor problems. There may be more gas, more disturbance and when we have more gas, what can we do? We have to neutralize the gas, so I suggest adding a good digestant. The digestant should be a whole digestant that takes care of starches, sugars and proteins. It is made of pancreatic substance and a little betaine hydrochloric acid. It is an all-around good digestant, but vegetarians might prefer to use the herbal digestants available. For vegetarians we recommend a substance called D&F, short for digestion and flatulence (gas), because we may begin to stir these up when we get into the bowel pockets.

I know of patients who began their diets and reported they had more gas than ever before. This is sometimes to be expected. Some people practically live on coffee and donuts, and they find they don't have gas, but they are worn out. They have no energy. You have to "rough it out" through this initial period of regeneration—this period of making new tissue—before your digestive system will normalize.

A certain amount of gas is normal for the average person. I don't believe anybody has a perfect bowel. I think a little gas will be produced by anyone, and every farmer knows that when you give a lot of fresh alfalfa to a horse he has more gas than usual. Is that horse getting worse? No, it is in better condition. We find that it has a better bowel. So I believe alfalfa tablets and the digestant are very important. We find that the acidophilus culture, given morning and evening, is an excellent way of developing good bacteria in the bowel.

At the Battle Creek Sanitarium, researchers found that meat was very detrimental to the bowel because it is very putrefactive. It is best to cut meat to a minimum in the diet and to upgrade the intake of vegetables. More greens will help to develop acidophilus bacteria. Chocolate, tea (not herb teas), white sugar and coffee break down acidophilus bacteria so we must eliminate or minimize the use of such substances. A successful bowel management program requires that we go a different way.

In following a program for the bowel, there are some excellent corrective exercises. There is an exercise to use on the slant board which involves vigorous tapping of the abdomen while stretching the upper torso from side to side. This exercise gently pulls the bowel down in the direction of the shoulders while upside-down on the board. I'm interested in getting the bowel in the proper position. I believe we have been crowding the bowel. So we must go to work on it. Doing the bicycle pedaling exercise while up-side down on the slant board is a wonderful exercise. For another type of exercise, lie down and take a rubber ball or tennis ball and rub it around in a circle on your abdomen. The round surface of the ball gets right down into the bowel and gives it an internal exercise, more so than rubbing on the outside. There are other exercises to lift the bowel and manipulate the prolapsus back into position.

SLANT BOARD EXERCISES
(For Prolapsus and Regenerating the Vital Nerve Centers of the Brain)

When there is a lack of tone in the muscles, we can expect prolapsus of the abdominal organs. The heart, lacking tone, cannot circulate blood properly throughout the body. Likewise, arteries and veins cannot contract to help the blood fight gravity and get into the brain tissues.

There are some people who apparently have tried everything to get well, who still find all organs working under par. Many people do not realize that the quickening force for every organ of the body comes from the brain. People whose occupations require them to sit or stand continually are unable to get the blood into the brain tissues because the tired organs cannot force the blood uphill. If we deny the brain tissues good blood in the proper amount, eventually every organ in our body will suffer.

The heart gets its start from the brain and continues its everlasting pumping because of it. No organ can do without the brain. I attribute the success of my healing work to the very fact that I definitely recognize that the brain must be fed properly. Slanting board exercises are absolutely necessary to regain perfect health.

CAUTIONARY NOTE

There are many cases where the board is contra-indicated. It is best in most cases to get professional advice, for some people have had unhappy experiences due to the very fact they started too strenuous a program to begin with. If you haven't done much exercising of the abdominal muscles, it is best to take these exercises slowly and gradually increase them as you get stronger.

Do not use the board in cases of high blood pressure, hemorrhages, some tubercular conditions, cancer in the pelvic cavity, appendicitis, ulcers of the stomach or intestines or pregnancy, unless under the care of a physician.

The slanting board exercises are practically the same as any other lying-down exercises. The most important exercise is to hold on to the sides of the board bringing the knees up to the chest. This forces all the abdominal organs up toward the shoulders. While in this position, twist the head from side to side and in all directions, thus utilizing the extra force to circulate blood to congested areas of the head, especially bringing the stomach and abdominal organs up toward the chest while holding the breath.

Slanting board exercises are especially good in cases of inflammations and congestions above the shoulders, such as sinus trouble, bad eyes, falling hair, head eczema, ear conditions and similar troubles. Slanting board exercise is needed and has helped more than any other treatment in cases of heart trouble, fatigue, dizziness, poor memory and paralysis. The average person should maintain the foot end of the board at chair height for all exercises, but if dizzy at first, the foot end of the board should not be raised quite so high. Exercise only 5 minutes a day. Gradually increase time spent on the board. The average patient should lie on the board 10 minutes at 3 o'clock in the afternoon and again just before going to bed. After retiring, lift the buttocks to allow the organs to return to a normal position.

SUGGESTED EXERCISES

(Use Ankle Straps While Doing the Following Exercises)

(Numbered exercises correspond to illustrations.)

1. Lie full length, allowing gravity to help the abdominal organs into their position. For best results, lie on board at least 10 minutes.

2. While lying flat on back, stretch the abdomen by putting arms above head. Bring arms above head 10 to 15 times; this stretches the abdominal muscles and pulls the abdomen down toward the shoulders.

3. Bring abdominal organs toward shoulders while holding breath. Move the organs back and forth by drawing them upward, contracting abdominal muscles, then allowing them to go back to a relaxed position. Do this 10 to 15 times.

4. Pat abdomen vigorously with open hands. Lean to one side then to the other, patting the stretched side. Pat 10 to 15 times each side.

   Bring the body to sitting position, using the abdominal muscles. Return to lying position. Do this 3 to 4 times, if possible. Do only if doctor orders.

HOLD ON TO THE HANDLES, FEET OUT OF STRAPS, WHILE DOING THESE EXERCISES:

5. Bend knees and legs at hips. While in this position: (a) turn head from side to side 5 or 6 times;   (b) lift head slightly and rotate in circles 3 or 4 times.

6. Lift legs to vertical position, rotate outward in circles 8 or 10 times. Increase to 25 times after a week or two of exercising.

7. Bring legs straight up to a vertical position and lower them to the board slowly. Repeat 3 or 4 times.

8. Bicycle legs in air 15 to 25 times.

   Relax and rest, letting the blood circulate in the head for 10 minutes.

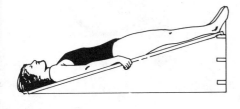

1

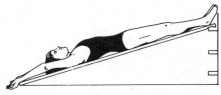

2

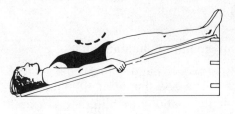

3

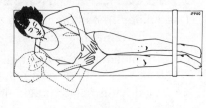

4

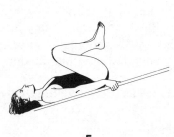

5

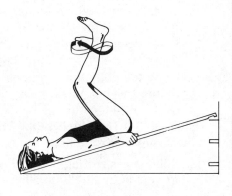

6

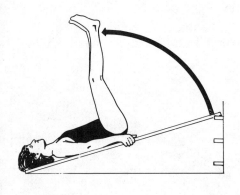

7

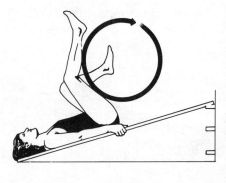

8

ELEVEN-DAY ELIMINATION REGIME

There are many eliminative regimes, and they all accomplish about the same results, through the fact that the body is given less food, simpler foods and simpler combinations, more watery foods—so a greater transition can take place in the cells of the body.

This Eleven-Day Elimination Regime can be used by most persons in health, and for those who want to overcome the average physical disorder. Those who are weak or feeble, however, should not follow the plan the full eleven days without supervision. Those with tuberculosis should have both supervision and assistance.

Variation, as to the length of time and the manner in which the foods are to be taken, may be adjusted to suit the history of the patient. Examples: fruits, vegetables and broths can be taken for 1 day; or 1 day of just fruit; or 1, 2 or 3 days of vegetables only.

Vegetables, taken in the form of broths, gently steamed vegetables and salads are a safer routine for the average beginner than citrus fruits.

A hot bath should be taken every night during this diet regime. Enemas may be used the first four or five days, then discontinued for natural movements. Nothing but water and fruit juices, preferably grapefruit, should be taken into the body for the first three days. Drink one glass of juice every four hours of the day. The next two days fruit only—such as grapes, melons, tomatoes, pears, peaches, plums; dried fruit such as prunes, figs, peaches, soaked overnight or baked apple.

In the six following days, breakfast should consist of citrus fruits. Between breakfast and lunch, any other kind of fruit. For lunch, have a salad of three to six vegetables and two cups of vital broth. When hungry between meals, fruit or fruit juices may be taken. Dinner should consist of two or three steamed vegetables and two cups of vital broth. Fruit juices can be taken before retiring, if wanted.

Rigid adherence to the diet is an absolute necessity for anyone attempting to regain good health. Eat plenty, but not to satiety.

VITAL BROTH RECIPE:

2 C. carrot tops; 1 clove garlic; 2 C. potato peelings (1/2" thick); 2 C. beet tops; 2 C. celery tops; 3 C. celery stalk; 2 qt distilled water; 1/2 tsp Savita or Vegex. Add a carrot and onion to flavor, if desired (grate or chop).

Ingredients should be finely chopped. Bring to a boil, slowly; simmer approximately 20 minutes. Use only the broth after straining.

When finished with the above regime return to Dr. Jensen's Daily Food Regime.

The above elimination regime should be followed whenever a person changes from the old ways of living and begins to live right. As a rule, it is wise to follow the elimination regime in any and all of the following cases: as a general cleanser two or three times a year; at the time of crisis; when reduction of weight is desired; when hips get too large; when joints get stiff; when the skin breaks out; when constipation is present.

THE MASTER CHLOROPHYLL ELIMINATION DIET

This is a diet of just plain water, preferably using distilled water, and using one teaspoon of a liquid chlorophyll to one glass of water every three hours. You can also use vegetable juice, but this is a diet where we are adding iron, gathering all the oxygen we can while we are breathing, and burning up the toxic waste by using the iron as found in liquid chlorophyll. Liquid chlorophyll is usually made as an extract from alfalfa leaves, which is one of the highest things we have in potassium iron, which will attract the oxygen to the body. Doing this for three or four days is a wonderful preelimination diet to fasting or to any other type of dieting. I consider this to be the master-cleansing diet for all catarrhal conditions. In the presence of greens, we find that catarrh is eliminated best from the body.

WATERMELON FLUSH

There are times during the watermelon season that we can use watermelon as a good elimination diet. Going on watermelon for three, four or five days is a wonderful kidney eliminant, a diuretic. We find that it helps to take out a lot of the debris in the colon and the extra water picks up toxic materials and carries them off.

ONE DAY A WEEK FAST

On a one day a week fast regime you can be on a juice diet or a fruit on the one day—and rest. Many people like to go on a fast one day a week. This is perfectly all right if you will rest that day—but you **MUST** rest! You cannot expect to get the good yielded by a rest without food by using all of your energy and leaving yourself depleted by working on a day that you do not eat.

FASTING

Fasting is the quickest way of bringing about elimination in the body and the fastest way of getting toxic materials out of the body. This is done through complete rest—physical, psychological and psychic.

As we let the body rest, it develops tone and vitality, more than is possible by any other procedure. I believe rest is a cure because it gives us the vitality we need to throw off toxic material and to eliminate the debris that has been accumulated over a period of years. We can literally withdraw toxic accumulations through a fast. We find that there are many ways to fast. I think the better way is to take a half glass of water every hour and a half throughout the day. If it is a hot day, you may need more water and it is all right since you perspire more. Be sure not to take big gulps of water at one time. The water should be cool but not ice cold.

Take daily enemas the first few days, then reduce this to every other day or every third or fourth day, depending upon the length of time you fast. While you are fasting you should rest as much as possible. If you hike or walk, do it on level ground. Do nothing to the point of tiring. This is important in fasting.

JUICE FASTING

I don't think it's any particular juice that will cure anything—but I believe the rest you give your body allows it the opportunity to reverse the disease and recover your health. It's the rest from food and the simple diet that does the trick. The lack of too many food mixtures and less demand made on our digestive and eliminative systems help us to overcome disease.

The carrot juice diet involves taking one glass of carrot juice every three hours or more if you like. You can do this for ten days, twenty days or even longer. I had one man on carrot juice for a whole year. That is a long time! This particular man lived in Monrovia and had an extreme condition of the bowel but through the carrot juice diet, he got rid of it.

Dr. Kirschner, who wrote the book on juice therapy, came here to talk over this man's case because he found out how I had kept him on juices for so long a time. The man passed off mucus and catarrh continually from that bowel. It was almost unbelievable what was eliminated—being even black at times. This was simply accumulated toxic material that was necessary for him to get rid of.

BREAKING A FAST

In breaking a fast, if you go five, six or seven days on water, then go one or two days on juices, either vegetable or fruit. Take one 8-oz glass every three hours. You have eliminated the enemas one or two days beforehand and you are starting in to work for good bowel movements now.

After the two days of juices, start the first thing in the morning on the third day with sliced or peeled oranges. The bulk of an orange is probably one of the finest things for the bowel. If you do not want to use oranges, you can use a finely shredded carrot that has been steamed or wilted for one minute. This acts to help clean out the toxic materials. You can do this for breakfast and lunch. Then for the evening meal, you can start out with a small salad.

Have a glass of juice at 10:00 am and again at 3:00 pm.

The next day you can have fresh fruit for breakfast along with juice. Have juice at 10:00 am. For lunch, you can have a small salad and juice. Have another glass of juice at 3:00 pm.

At the evening meal you can have a salad, one cooked vegetable and juice.

The next day you can have the same as the day before, except that you could have an extra vegetable at noon and again at night, if desired. You may also have an egg or a tablespoon of nut butter for the morning meal.

The next day, you will start on Dr. Jensen's Regular Diet, except for no starches.

The day following, you can have both starches and proteins in your diet.

NOTE

Here is a simple thing for you to remember when considering the basic requirements for good bowel management. Your food should in some way contribute to the BLM in the bowel. BLM is Bulk, Lubrication and Moisture. These three combine to provide an ideal bowel environment. Bulk creates the mass whereby good evacuation is assured. Lubrication provides an easy flow of materials through the digestive tract *all* the way to the anus. Moisture prevents the drying out of feces and constipation from developing. If your food item does not contribute to BLM, then don't eat it!

GRAPES

Four pounds of grapes a day is a good amount for a grape diet and you should average a pound or so every three hours. These grapes should be the grapes that have seeds since these are the most vital of all grapes. Man has gone to using hybrid foods too much. Those foods that were brought to us in the beginning are the foods that have lots of seeds. They are the vital foods. So I believe the grapes that have seeds are the best. The Concord, Fresno Beauty, Red grapes and Muscat, all are good grapes to use. I don't say that you have to use the seeds. You can chew them finely if you like. A good thing to help eliminate catarrh is found in cream of tartar which surround the seeds. So make sure you get all the material off the seeds when you are eating them. When chewing grape skins, you'll find that they are very bitter but that bitterness is high in potassium. Potassium is a great cleanser in the body. Gayelord Hauser made his name with potassium broth. It is a great cleanser and detoxifier in the body.

Especially in the beginning of the grape diet, I think you should use enemas. Toxic materials accumulate and it is well that we keep things moving along. You can go on grapes five to ten days without any supervision, but if you stay on them longer, it is well to have someone around who has been used to giving the grape diet. That person should be able to take care of you with any reaction you might have that may be strange to you. Many times these reactions are nothing more than a healing crisis or an elimination process.

WATER REMEDIES

Sitz Baths. Water should come up five inches on the body. The feet are never in the water. The baths should only be for the pelvis and the pelvic organs. This is wonderful for congestion in the pelvis and sluggish bowels. These baths are best taken in the evening just before going to bed. However, they can be taken the first thing in the morning before going to work.

The cold sitz bath is an effective, though violent way of stopping bedwetting. Take cold water, sitting in it four to five minutes every morning before going to school or before beginning the daily program or routine. This will help with bladder and prostate, problems in general. A gentler approach is to take two sitz baths every morning. The first for one minute, hot; the second for one-half minute, cold. Do this for five changes, going from one to the other. The treatment should continue for a period of three months.

BENEFITS OF THE ENEMA

Enemas can be beneficial in restoring healthy bowel regularity. This is why I believe enemas should be used every day for a year by those who have problems with a sluggish, irregular or underactive bowel. Many ingredients can be added to enema water to increase its effectiveness in some specific manner. Coffee enemas help detoxify the liver. Flaxseed tea enemas relieve inflammation in the bowel. Bentonite, a clay water, when added to enema water assists in absorbing and mobilizing toxins from the bowel wall. Acidophilus culture taken orally is helpful in detoxifying the bowel and in building friendly bacteria. Acidophilus implants can also be inserted rectally over night.

I believe that each of the many health professions and approaches to health care have a special value. I do not believe, however, that any therapeutic method—no matter how sophisticated—can effectively overcome disease in a toxic-laden body. The toxins must be eliminated first. Nor do I believe that any drug-based therapy can restore or rejuvenate tissue damaged in the course of chronic disease. Only nutrients from foods can do that. I believe when we work with nature, we get the results nature intends us to get. A clean body nourished by natural foods and uplifting thoughts will put anyone on the path to right living that brings health as a natural consequence.

It is interesting to note that the famous beauty queen, whom I knew, Mae West, was a great believer in the benefits of the enema. She started every day with a morning enema. I'm sure that this simple practice greatly contributed to her unusual vitality, bright mindedness and long lasting attractiveness, as true beauty is but a reflection of the beauty within.

A WORD ABOUT COLONICS

Colonics, as administered today, vary greatly in their effects due largely to the expertise of the colonic technician.

We feel that in some respects colonic therapy is taking advantage of people by making them believe that long and costly treatments are necessary. Also water applied under pressure is potentially hazardous. Those individuals with known or suspected serious bowel problems should approach pressurized colonic treatments with extreme caution.

Those practitioners who administer colonic therapy properly are offering a useful service to the public. This service can be greatly enhanced with the addition of sound dietary counseling so as to eventually overcome the need for colonic therapy. Without this knowledge, the colonic recipient is merely digging holes and filling them again—a net zero toward building a better health quality.

Many professionals giving colonics today are getting successful but temporary results. The reason for this is that just getting rid of the toxic waste in the bowel is not the complete answer, although it is the first step along the correct path. Unless proper exercise, diet and right living are practiced, good and lasting results will not be achieved. We must be interested in making bowel tissue changes.

REVITALIZING BROTH

This is a broth that was used during my sanitarium work dealing with very sick people who had to be nourished back to health. It is very easy to digest.

Use 5 or 6 of these non-gas-forming vegetables, such as: Beets, carrots, potato peeling, celery, parsley, okra (if possible), chayote pear or any squash.

Do not use any of the sulfur vegetables: cabbage, cauliflower, broccoli or onions.

Add: 1 C. cut up vegetables; 1 pint water; 2 tablespoons Soybean Milk Powder.

After either liquifying, blending or shredding vegetables, place in a pot with other ingredients and let simmer 3-5 minutes over a very low flame.

This is only to break down the fiber and release enzymes. Strain and use.

Chapter 8

INTRODUCTION TO THE ULTIMATE TISSUE CLEANSING SYSTEM

I've given colonics to people who have expelled grape seeds and they had not eaten grapes for nine months! Where had those seeds been? I've seen popcorn come out of a person when they hadn't had popcorn for three years. Where had it been? We accumulate these things in the mucous membrane that holds toxic material in various folds of the intestines. It was very hard for me to believe this could happen.

Just a short time ago, I went through the Ultimate Cleansing process, and I can attest to the wonderful results I experienced. For those who have asthma, an extreme elimination program will help you more than anything; and for those who suffer with arthritis, I have seen many receive relief within ten days after participating in this program. I can tell you about cases and relief that came to those who have taken care of the bowel. It is a means of keeping the body clean. *"Cleanse and purify thyself and I will exalt thee to the throne of power."* Energy which flows through our body is dependent upon a clean body.

For example, here is a case that was quite striking to me. One of the women on the program who is in her early fifties, had medical laboratory tests taken that showed a triglyceride reading of 938 mg/dl (Normal is 150-200.) and a cholesterol reading of 348 mg/dl. After one week on the Ultimate Cleansing Program, the triglyceride dropped to 253 and the cholesterol to 277; obviously a dramatic change occurred.

There is a mucous membrane that lines the last six feet of the intestinal tract of the large colon. I never believed this tract could be so mucus loaded, black and toxic, but I had the chance to see this while on the Ultimate Cleansing Program myself. In this process, you use an intestinal bulk. This bulk is mixed with clay water and is taken five times a day followed by a second drink of natural apple cider vinegar and honey. Hot water carries food or any material to the colon, while cold water and food stop at the stomach. This is why we do not believe in cold food or drinks after meals; this stops digestive processes at the stomach level. We find that hot drinks will get to the bowel and start things moving along. The instructions for the 7-day cleansing program are more detailed in the next section.

Now there are ways of breaking down the mucous membrane. How did you happen to get this heavy mucous membrane? You were not digesting your foods properly. In those who don't digest food properly, the pancreas isn't working well, so they can get relief by taking Pancreatic tablets. Most of this heavy mucus, I believe, has been developed by undigested foods. By putting this excess amount of pancreatic material in the body, you can readjust what the pancreas should have done in the past when the body was overloaded with starches, sugar, etc. We are now going to readjust this so it will tear down the mucus that holds all of these materials. I believe the digestant will also help break off the mucous lining from the bowel wall. I believe this because I've been on several elimination programs and this one rids the bowel of the mucous lining.

When the liver hasn't been working too well and we are a wee bit on the slow side in moving the bowel, it may help to take beet tablets. Further, we may want to take Spring Green or Green Life tablets. No food will be eaten during this time. You have only a small amount of juice mixed with the bulk and the rest is water. The vitamins and minerals in tablet form are all food, so you won't feel hungry. You won't lose much weight on your first cleansing elimination.

There are more vitamins and minerals to take and I think one to be considered is niacin. This pushes blood to all the different organs in the body. Niacin will give you a hot flash and a flush; we want the blood to get to the bowel wall at this time.

There is a product called Calphonite which is colloidal calcium and is taken twice a day, morning and night. At night, cod liver oil is added which will control and fix calcium in the body. Calphonite is a refined lime product with a very high absorption rate which promotes the dissolving of precipitated calcium settled in the joints.

THE CLEANSING PROGRAM

I would like to discuss one of the most important aspects of the bowel management program, the one most neglected and the one no one wants to talk about. I think we are all in a bowel mess because we grew up like Topsy, and now we have to talk about it. We have to begin to correct old errors by learning the right way to take care of the bowel.

Cleansing, detoxification and elimination are words we all hear, but they are seldom used in connection with the bowel. When I look over all the programs that were developed to take care of the bowel and all the various techniques we've had in bowel cleansing, I have come to the conclusion that a real cleansing process should be one that reaches every cell in the body. In general, we can say that the blood is only as clean as the bowel, and since the blood circulates through every organ in the body and reaches every cell in the body, toxins in the blood due to a dirty bowel contaminate the entire body. To properly cleanse the body tissue we must start by a thorough cleansing of the bowel.

We have to utilize energy to rid the bowel of toxic material. We find, too, that the bowel has to take care of acids. Catarrh elimination through the bowel is actually part of our own body being eliminated. Now, I've heard the bowel called a cesspool and I've heard it called the dirtiest part of the body. I point this out because the average person doesn't want to talk about it; such discussion is thought to be socially unacceptable. Bowel problems should be discussed, however, because most people need some help. There is nothing to be ashamed of in discussing the bowel. It is merely a natural part of the body. Care of the bowel should be a routine part of a total health program.

Bowel action is one of the end results of metabolism; the elimination of broken down cells and tissue plus the fermented and putrified food wastes. Bowel action is far worse when there is a lazy colon. The colon is made up of muscle structure that moves toxic materials along by peristaltic motion, and if there is flabby muscle structure throughout the body, you can be assured that the bowel is even flabbier.

"IT'S NOT ONLY WHAT YOU EAT—IT'S WHAT YOU ABSORB THAT COUNTS"

In managing the bowel, there are ways to get good results, and first of all, we must change the diet. Unless we do this, we will become "doctor shoppers." The symptoms just stay with us because we aren't dealing with the cause of the problem. Every organ in the body works with every other organ. The body is a community of various organs working for the good of the whole human being.

A short word on intestinal cultures before the story. While I was at the Battle Creek Sanitarium, Dr. DeFoe, who delivered the famous Dionne quintuplets in Canada, telephoned Dr. John Harvey Kellogg and said he was about to lose two of the babies because of their poor bowel conditions. Dr. Kellogg immediately sent off an acidophilus culture, and a week later, Dr. DeFoe called to say the two babies were much improved. He felt that Dr. Kellogg had saved the babies' lives with the acidophilus culture.

In discussing the many types of diets that are appropriate during the different stages of disease, we must be sensitive to what these stages represent in terms of digestive ability.

For instance, we can't immediately give a big raw salad to one who has colitis; we must first cleanse and give the bowel tonicity in preparation for more efficient digestion and absorption.

Going through the 7-day elimination program will give us a head start. We must be able to absorb the nutrients that we are rebuilding our bodies with or those nutrients will be lost.

Once absorption has been increased we take the body step by step along a graduated food regime. We may have to use broths and light soups at first, then go on to steamed, pureed vegetables and fruits. Raw, liquefied salads can be given as the bowel becomes able to handle more bulk.

We must move slowly but surely along the tissue cleansing and rejuvenating system, keeping in mind that even as it took time to pollute our bodies to the point of disease, so it will take time to reverse the process.

POOR ASSIMILATION LEADS TO NUTRITIONAL DEFICIENCIES

Personally, I wonder if a toxic body can even absorb the right chemical elements at all. If body tissue is unable to function at the normal metabolic rate, regeneration and rebuilding would take a great deal longer than otherwise. Can digestion be good in a toxic body? It is impossible to build healthy tissue without effective digestion and assimilation.

Nerve conduction is not as effective as it should be when the metabolic rate is low. It is entirely possible to have good nerve flow and nerve function in the body, but if the body chemistry is not right, improvement through rejuvenation will be limited and incomplete. A complete tissue detoxification program requires that we take care of all five elimination channels. Underactive tissue cannot get rid of toxic wastes properly. I want to place a special emphasis on this. When we rid the body of toxins, we often notice a subsequent remission of some degenerative disease stage.

CLEAN TISSUES FUNCTION BETTER

There are many therapeutic approaches to restoring or maintaining health today. However, the presence of toxic settlements in the body prevents any of these methods of treatment from being completely successful. If a treatment does not work toward complete detoxification, the rejuvenation of tissue will not take place as it should. The complete rejuvenation process involves the replacement of old underactive tissue with new, clean, efficiently working tissue. This is what brings a degenerative condition to a state of recession and remission. Many kinds of processes can be used to bring this about, and this is what the doctor must be alert for.

The natural immune system can only be built up in a clean body, a body with a minimal amount of accumulated toxic material. The presence of significant quantities of toxic material in body tissue means that the body's natural defenses have been overcome. When health is restored through a tissue cleansing program, the immune system will also be restored as we return to a healthy diet, exercise, fresh air, sunshine and a positive outlook on life.

Most people believe that tissue rebuilding depends upon a nutritious diet, and this is basically correct. But it also depends on good nerve force, good circulation and adequate rest.

We have done experiments to show what can be accomplished by tissue detoxification. In a period of only seven days of fasting, taking nutritional supplements and bowel cleansing, almost unbelievable results have been observed and recorded. As these methods are further understood and tested; we may hope to find them in hospitals and sanitariums in the treatment of disease.

In order to reverse the disease process, we must consider Hering's law of cure, which states that all diseases are cured from within out, from the head down and in reverse order as their symptoms first appeared in the body. This means we have to return over the same "track" we traveled to get the disease. No disease can exist without toxic material in the body, so the first step toward remission is detoxification.

To administer drugs in response to a disease condition brought on by toxic accumulations can only add to the problem. Although temporary relief may be obtained, the residual drug settlement will, over the long term, simply increase the toxic burden of the body.

Please remember that this program is designed to be part of a preventive health care system in which the results of bad habits may begin to be reversed. No good results of lasting quality will be had as long as destructive habits are continued. This program is for the person who is wanting and willing to start over anew. Taking up the life-generating practices marks the beginning of a new day toward the harvest of renewed health and vitality.

Throughout this book, we have stressed the importance of cleanliness as the vehicle by which health is regained and maintained. The degree to which the colon is inhabited by harmful bacteria, parasites and other dangerous organisms varies greatly among individuals. What one person is able to hold in the bowel without obvious effects may be hazardous to others.

❖ *SANITATION & CLEANLINESS IMPORTANT NOTE* ❖

Contamination by one individual of another must be avoided. *This important point is best accomplished by each person having their own personal colema board and tip.* **DO NOT ALLOW ANOTHER PERSON TO USE YOUR BOARD OR TIP UNLESS THE EQUIPMENT HAS BEEN COMPLETELY STERILIZED.** *Microscopic organisms are very easily transferred to the colon by the use of unclean colema rectal tips. Store your rectal tip in a bottle of germicidal solution when not in use. Sterilize the interior tube to which the rectal tube is attached before use to ensure against infection. We have endeavored to make this system as easy as possible to keep clean by making it simple and uncomplicated. Thorough cleansing of the board after each use is essential to avoiding complications. It is very important that this instruction be adhered to for your health and well-being.* **Do not be lax in this regard.**

One of the nice advantages of this system is that colonic debris never flows back through the colema tubing, as occurs in nearly all commercially available colonic irrigation equipment. In this way, contamination is kept to a safe minimum. It is a good idea to occasionally cleanse the hoses of the colema by running a germicidal solution through the bucket and tubing to cleanse the passageways of any possible infestations. Also, always keep a protective lid on the colema bucket to avoid settlement of hair, dust, dirt or other contamination into the bucket. Always thoroughly rinse the bucket before and after each use.

Another important consideration that you should be aware of is the quality of your water supply. Contaminated water can cause severe bowel distress. If you are working with well water in your colema, it is a good idea to make certain the water is safe for colonic irrigation by having it tested at your local health certification agency. If in doubt, it is suggested you take measures to sterilize the water by some means such as boiling or passing it through an antibacterial filtration. Chemical treatment should not be used unless there is no other choice. Chlorine, such as bleaching agents, will sterilize water but is unfit to use immediately. If chlorinated water is used, it should be allowed to stand vented overnight so the chlorine vapors dissipate. There should be little or no chlorine residue left in the water when it is used for the colema treatment.

It is possible that your water supply is irritating to your bowel. To help solve this problem, we suggest that flaxseed tea be used. Flaxseed tea, as prepared on page 109, is a very soothing, healing and lubricating substance when added to the colema water solution.

THE ULTIMATE TISSUE CLEANSING SYSTEM

Unlike Any Other System in Cleansing and Regenerating the Body!

ACKNOWLEDGMENT

Bowel cleansing and healthy bowel management has been studied extensively by Mr. V. E. Irons. Mr. Irons is a leading specialist on bowel problems, and for 42 years he has endeavored to understand the workings and needs of the healthy bowel. He heads the V. E. Irons Company of Natick, Massachusetts, where VIT-RA-TOX products are distributed. He is a leading advocate in the use of natural substances, believing strongly that the body is fully capable of healing itself when given the opportunity. His experience has shown that very few people have normal bowel function.

Mr. Irons and I have been working together for many years and see eye to eye that the bowel is the basis for most of humanity's ailments today. While it is necesary to take care of the bowel it is only one aspect that must be cared for to bring on perfect health. We consider Mr. V. E. Irons to be one of our best friends. He is one I am indebted to for the ideas worked out in this colema program. After many years of using this, we consider this program to be the fastest, easiest and least complicated tissue cleansing program available today. One important point to remember, however, is that some people cannot go through the whole 7-day program. The seriously ill patient or the elderly may only be able to go on this program for one day.

Kay Shaffer has contributed much time, effort and creative energy into developing this program.

She is a tireless worker in bowel cleansing-management and has worked with Mr. Irons for many years. She has had outstanding results and has seen some of the most unbelievable symptoms reverse as a result of this treatment.

Sylvia Bell has coauthored this book with me and has worked consistently on all the treatments we have given at our Ranch-Sanitarium. She has assisted greatly in bringing this work forward.

OUR GOAL

The following information is a step-by-step, detailed instruction on the procedure and operation of the Ultimate Tissue Cleansing System as it is used at the writing of this book.

We endeavor to employ the most thorough, efficient and natural means available toward the goal of tissue detoxification and cleansing. Therefore, ongoing research and development are in progress toward this end.

Our goal is to serve humanity by exploring and revealing those methods, products, procedures and creative insights as they are presented to us for the express purpose of relieving pain, suffering, disease and premature aging.

We strive to learn the ways to reinstate the natural, God-given gifts of health, vitality and longevity to those who seek them in these days of unprecedented toxic pollution.

During the many years of helping people correct poor bowel conditions, it has become very obvious that most people are not capable of taking good care of themselves.

There is no reason to be afraid of this treatment because it is safe, gentle and comfortable on the body. There is nothing mysterious about its workings and anyone who can read and follow simple instructions can do this work for themselves.

On a limited basis, we conduct classes and training for this treatment. At the moment, we are working with a seven-day experimental live-in program designed to give practitioners a first-hand experience of the system in action. Write for details.

I am convinced that this treatment makes nutrients available to the body faster than any other system I know of, because the bowel is cleaner and the colon muscle tone is stronger. When the bowel is toxic laden, it becomes lazy, loses its ability to function in all capacities and soon loses its muscle tone.

It takes an internal manipulation to restore good bowel function once it is lost. The colema treatment does this work because it is an internal massage which develops muscular tone in the bowel. It takes a year to build good tone by this method. I don't know of any other system that can give you these results any quicker.

Compared to other treatments, this ultimate tissue cleansing system is exceptionally cost effective, making it within reach for a great many people.

I want to make this system of cleansing and healing available to everyone and this is the main reason for this book. Whether it is handed to someone in the wilds of Canada or the jungles of South America, they should be able to understand this book and go through this treatment to help overcome disease and illness.

With this system of tissue cleansing, we're going to take the buildup of mucus and catarrh which has become sticky, congested and hardened, and liquify it so that it will run out of the body. This is the beginning of the program.

The real work in healing the body is going to come later when there is a transformation in tissue integrity resulting in a higher quality body. This process brings on the healing crisis and may take 6 months to bring on a complete elimination. This will result in cleaner, purer tissue that is able to accept and handle the good, vital foods you're feeding it.

This program is not just a colonic—it is much more. We call it a colema because it's a combination of an enema and a colonic.

This program involves more than just taking care of the bowel. We must prepare the body's elimination channels for the housecleaning that is on the way. If we build the body up to cause a cleansing to occur, then we must open up the elimination systems to handle this discarded material. It is common for old, toxic substances to flow not only from the bowel, but from all channels; lungs, mouth, nose, ears, skin, kidneys, lymph, vagina; all possible channels must be ready and capable of handling the flood.

In preparing for this occurrence, I strongly advise that you become more familiar with the process by studying my book which explains the healing crisis in detail, titled *Doctor-Patient Handbook*.

One of the usual occurrences for those who have experienced this system is the extreme elimination of feces. One patient explains that she could have a complete bowel movement and then take a colema and have still another bowel movement and, after an hour or so, have another complete bowel movement!

Many people think that they are cleaned out when they have one movement. Unfortunately, most people are as many as 10 meals behind in their eliminations! They are holding many meals in the ballooning, pocketed portions of their bowel.

The colema treatment will loosen up this material and make it flow. It will also restore tone and activity to that part of the bowel that is distorted and underactive.

We've had some people who are afraid that they are losing part of the bowel because the material coming through is so unbelievable in its shape, color, consistency and odor. They can't imagine the heavy mucous lining being so foul, thick and stringy.

This is not a desirable thing to retain in the bowel because it is carrying the seeds of disease and illness. It is loaded with old drugs, tissue and morbid substances. It is the favored environment for the disease-producing bacillus coli.

As the body rises up from the old, we must work with it, support it and encourage the process. We work with less food, more broths, more rest. The body responds with revitalization and regeneration in all the tissues of the organism.

This is why we call it a tissue cleansing treatment. It gets after every tissue in the body, not just the bowel. We realize by now that every tissue in the body is as clean as the bowel. This is due to the fact that every tissue is fed by the blood which is nourished by the bowel. When the bowel is dirty, the blood is dirty and so on to the organs and tissues.

When diarrhea comes along, don't stop it. Let it go, it is a cleansing process. Drink plenty of liquids to avoid being dehydrated. During the healing crisis, do not eat very much; nothing at all is best. Overeating during this time will possibly shut down the process and thereby delay that which you have worked so hard to make occur.

Go instead to the vegetable juices, vegetable broths and light liquids. If there is any fever, do not use any fruit juices, especially citrus juices. Potato peeling broth is the best thing to use at this time. A fever indicates that the body is hard at work burning up toxic substances. Let's not interfere with it by forcing the body to divert needed cleansing energy into having to process food.

The bowel is like a vacuum cleaner bag. It filters and filters until it is all clogged up and doesn't do its job anymore. In fact, a clogged up bag causes damage to the motor by allowing debris to pass by where it finds its way into the delicate machinery. It also places a very heavy load upon the motor, which is trying to draw air through the dirty bag. The colema treatment unplugs the filter, so to speak.

This treatment will be relatively new to a lot of people. It can be used by young and old alike, as well as so-called healthy people. Practically any disease, discharging, infection, catarrhal or bowel disturbance and lowered hormone balance due to toxins can benefit from this treatment.

WHERE CAUTION IS NECESSARY

In diverticulitis we find that there can be severe reactions resulting from the painful condition that already exists in the patient. There may be abscesses forming. We might have a perforation of the bowel and we must be very careful in taking care of this. It will always be best to have a doctor's counsel and to see just what is going on. We find that if we can cleanse the bowel without any distention, even though using large amounts of water in the enema, we will be helping these sensitive problems.

We feel that the colema, which is one of the most natural ways of putting water into the bowel and eliminating it without any heavy distention, is probably the best way to take care of these things. However, we must make sure that we don't have any symptoms that are really grievous to the patient, mentally or physically. We must also watch that the white cell count does not become very high because we find that this will be a sign of infection and possibly conditions developing other than the diverticulitis that could be of a serious nature.

Further, we have to consider that there could be obstructions in that bowel from a growth and that to expect anything to happen immediately from the colema and from the tissue cleansing treatment may be unrealistic. It is always best to have a doctor check over these conditions to make sure this treatment can be used in combination with his suggestions and with his diagnosis.

WARNING AND ADVICE

Due to the fact that this can be considered the most powerful tissue cleansing treatment available today, some skill must be attended to persons given this treatment.

It is well to have the cooperation of a doctor to handle the most severe cases. It is also advisable to have a complete clinical examination so that all and any tests can be monitored as patient makes progress. This is not to be considered a "cure-all," but an adjunctive treatment. It is a foundation for thorough tissue detoxification by way of colon cleansing.

It is well to have complete regulatory and competent advisory consultation with those giving and administering this treatment.

A doctor knowing the "reversal process of cure" is to be desired. A disease in its reversal system will bring about different symptoms and can be responsible for elimination processes. Chemical, mechanical or nutritional assistance is also desirable and can be used with any other form of treatment favoring elimination and detoxification.

A clinical examination should basically include: urinalysis, a complete blood count, PBI, SMA-24, acid-alkaline fecal test, test for acidophilus bacteria, **X-rays when needed,** and any other test(s) that can be used to show tissue or functional changes taking place during this treatment. **Any particular weakness of any organ or system that is underactive should be tested often, or as deemed appropriate by doctor in order to monitor the patient closely.**

WARNING. Diabetic, tubercular, cancer and extreme degenerative diseases must have guidance, sanction and assistance by the most capable minds and doctor.

Diabetic cases must be handled with particular care in regard to the fasting aspect of the cleanse. Also all cases are not alike in their response to the detoxification program. Results may vary considerably according to individual constitutions.

Frequent colonic irrigation will have an adverse affect upon the electrolyte balance of the colon. Electrolyte leaching is not a good process and must be avoided. The best way to prevent this occurrence is to be absolutely certain that adequate amounts of lactobacillus organisms are reestablished in the colon. To accomplish this task, refer to pages 71 through 76 in this book. When the body is properly fed with good quality foods containing organic sodium, potassium and magnesium, the electrolyte level of the colon will be replenished as part of the diet. We must eat properly along with colon treatments. **DO NOT OVERLOOK THIS VERY IMPORTANT ASPECT OF COLON HEALTH.**

SUPPLEMENTS

A DEFINITION OF PROPERTIES

The following ingredients are used in the treatment for specific reasons. So that you may more fully appreciate the usefulness of these items, a brief explanation of their properties is included.

Alfalfa—The difference between alfalfa tablets, Green Life and Sun Chlorella is that alfalfa has all the fiber material left it it from the stems and fiber structure of the leaves. These act as a bulk and a material for a ballooned or weakened bowel to work against the tone of the tissues of the bowel. This also allows a faster transit time for the bowel. This is one of the supplements I use for practically every patient who needs to overcome bowel disturbances. Alfalfa offers the proper bulk, but sometimes produces more gas as we stir up this lazy bowel to act, and, for this reason, we use a couple of digestive enzymes to get rid of the gas.

Apple Juice—Very good for the bowel because it is high in pectin, which is a moisture-holding substance.

Apple Cider Vinegar—Very high in potassium and is good to relieve any mucus or catarrhal conditions. It helps provide needed nutrients to muscle tissue.

Beet Tablets—A slight laxative that works well with the liver, promoting the cleansing of that organ.

Bentonite—A clay suspended in water. It is very useful in absorbing toxic substances. It can absorb 40 times its own weight in toxic substances. It acts like a sponge, mopping up undesirable debris.

Mucilaginous Bulk—This material holds moisture well and attaches itself to the mucus lining making it soft and loose so it will move away from the bowel wall. This is a very important ingredient to the success of the treatment.

Cod Liver Oil—Provides lubrication and helps work with the liver in cleansing. It provides vitamins A and D which are needed for good elimination.

Coffee—Stimulates peristaltic action in the bowel—driving down feces and stimulating bile production in the liver.

Dulse—Quickens the thyroid gland and speeds up the metabolism while bringing heat to the body causing the blood to circulate deeper.

Spring Green and Green Life Tablets—Brand names for very potent biogenic plant substances. They provide rich sources of vitamins, minerals and enzymes that help in the cleansing process. We believe that Green Life is the finest supplements to be used with this colema program; however, if it is not available, you may use Sun Chlorella, in the same amount. Be sure to crush the tablets into powder form before taking.

Flaxseed—Excellent bulk maker, and in extreme cases of ulcerated colitis, provides a soothing and healing tea to be put into the colema water. It also is a bowel lubricant. For one of the colema solutions to be used when any serious cases are confronted, such as colitis, always use flaxseed tea. You can also add a teaspoon or more of liquid chlorophyll to this flaxseed tea for the colema water. This can be taken by mouth as well. When taken orally, use one cup tea and one teaspoon liquid chlorophyll three times a day. This can be used in cases of extreme gas, spastic conditions, colitis, etc.

Liquid Chlorophyll—Very wonderful for the bowel. It is soothing and reduces inflammation, swelling and pain. It disinfects and cleanses.

Niacin—Produces hot, red flush and is used to push the blood deep into underactive tissues so that we can strengthen them with vital nutritents.

Pancreatin—This is the one thing that helps most to bring down the mucus lining. It is a powerful digestant substance and loosens the lining.

Mr. Irons produces most of these products and they are very good. Nature's Sunshine is also producing similar products.

Please inquire for a very good all-around vitamin which is chemically balanced for both the adult and children.

I have had many requests from strict vegetarians about the use of the animal products in this treatment. Specifically, the Pancreatin and Cod Liver Oil. For those so concerned, I wish it were possible to recommend substitutes that are as effective as these. Unfortunately, I am not aware of any at this time. It is particularly important to use the Pancreatin as it has the unique ability to dissolve and digest the heavy mucus encrustation that causes so much of the bowel troubles.

Vitamin A is not readily available in a natural form other than cod liver oil. There are synthetic forms available, but I do not recommend their use. Vegetarian A is usually a pro-vitamin A and of low potency.

I feel that the benefits of this treatment outweight the use of the animal products for the brief period that they are employed. Once the bowel is reestablished into a healthier condition, then use of these substances can be discontinued.

Betaine HCL and herbal digestants have not given good results and are not recommended as viable substitutes for Pancreatin. Papaya tea or extract help. Huckleberry tea or extract may also be a substitute. We have not tried these and therefore cannot report on the effectiveness of them. If you suffer from an allergic reaction to any particular ingredient, then omit it from the program until it may be tolerated at a later time.

You will need:

1. Two empty pint jars with tight covers.
2. Juice. (Your choice of fruit juice. Apple is preferred or vegetable juice or natural herb teas for a variety of special purposes.)
3. 10 ounces of intestinal bulk; or like amount of ground psyllium seeds. Also needed: 8 herbal laxative tablets or equivalent.
4. Two bottle Bentonite clay water, Veico 77, VIT-RA-TOX 16, Sonne 7, Nature's Sunshine. (More needed if used in enema.)
5. Two bottles Spring Green or Green Life tablets preferred or liquid chlorophyll or eight alfalfa tablets.
6. One bottle wheat germ oil capsules.
7. One bottle vitamin C, 100 mg tablets.
8. One bottle beet juice tablets.
9. Colema board or enema bag with a long colonic tip (size 24 to 30, which is available at your drugstore). However, for the best results, a colema board is imperative.
10. One infant rectal syringe.
11. Calphonite or a calcium supplement like bone meal, etc.
12. Garlic capsules (used for certain conditions).
13. One quart apple cider vinegar (natural).
14. One pint honey.
15. Niacin (50-mg tablets).
16. Pancreatin tablets, quadruple strength, KAL brand or others.
17. Dulse tablets.
18. Cod liver oil, 1 pint—nonsynthetic, Norwegian cod is best.
19. Flaxseed, 8 ounces.
20. Coffee, ground (1 pound)—**not** instant coffee.
21. Rectal ointment: K-Y Jelly.

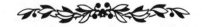

USE EXTREME CAUTION

Due to several complaints from colema users, we find it necessary to insist in the strongest possible language that ANY COLEMA TIP MUST NOT BE iNSERTED MORE THAN THREE (3) INCHES PAST THE ANUS WHEN TAKING COLEMAS. The bowel bends at the sigmoid flexure, about four (4) inches from the anus in the average person, perhaps less in some individuals. INSERTING ANY TIP MORE THAN THREE INCHES COULD BRING EXCESSIVE PRESSURE AGAINST THE BOWEL WALL AT THIS BEND, RESULTING IN IRRITATION, PAIN AND POSSIBLE MECHANICAL PROBLEMS. THERE SHOULD NEVER BE ANY FORCE EXERTED ON THE BOWEL WALL WITH ANY COLEMA TIP. This is another reason why we urge that our 7-DAY TISSUE CLEANSING PROGRAM be taken under the supervision of a doctor, colonic specialist or one versed in the proper use of enemas.

USE EXTREME CAUTION

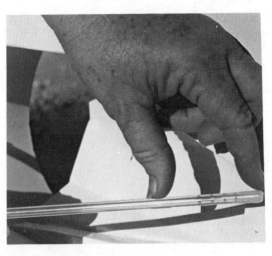

This illustration indicates 3 inches only on the tip which is to be inserted into the rectum.

7-DAY CLEANSING PROGRAM SCHEDULE

Eat **NOTHING** for the full 7 days, other than as specified, during the program. If you experience a feeling of extreme hunger, you may drink herbal teas, clear vegetable or potato peeling broths or diluted fresh vegetable juices. Plenty of liquid is essential to the success of the cleansing program.

The evening before starting the program, take 2 herbal laxative tablets. To ensure a more thorough elimination, use a baby enema syringe to inject 1 cup olive oil into rectum and hold until morning. If necessary in the morning, use an enema to make sure the lower colon is clean.

SKIN BRUSH
(Instructions on page 134) Your daily regimen should begin with skin brushing, 3 to 5 minutes.

CLEANSING DRINK
The cleansing drink consists of two parts to be mixed separately and drunk in succession. The two-part drink will be taken five times daily.

RECIPE

Part One:

2 oz Apple Juice
8 oz. water
1 tablespoon clay water
1 slightly rounded teaspoon intestinal cleanser
SHAKE WELL AND DRINK QUICKLY (mixture thickens).

Part Two:

10 oz. water
1 tablespoon Apple Cider Vinegar
1 teaspoon honey

SUPPLEMENTS

It is easiest to prepare the whole day's supplements at the beginning of each day. The supplements are to be taken 4 times each day. Separate them into 4 containers, one for each interval. See schedule for appropriate times. There will be different proportions on days One, Two and Three. Day Three through Seven will be the same.

The following supplements are taken in one interval. The *daily* intake will be 4 times this amount.

DAY ONE:

Green Life	12 each time
Niacin	50 mg each time
Wheat Germ Oil	1 capsule each time
Vitamin C	100 mg, 2 tablets each time
Pancreatin tablets	6 each time
Beet tablets	2 each time
Dulse tablets	1 each time

DAY TWO:

Green Life	18 each time
Niacin	100 mg each time
Wheat Germ Oil	1 capsule each time
Vitamin C	100 mg, 2 tablets each time
Pancreatin tablets	6 each time
Beet tablets	2 each time
Dulse tablets	1 each time

DAY THREE-SEVEN:

Green Life	24 each time
Niacin	150 mg up to 200 mg each time
Wheat Germ Oil	1 capsule each time
Vitamin C	100 mg, 3 tablets each time
Pancreatin tablets	6 each time
Beet tablets	2 each time
Dulse tablets	1 each time

Along with the pill supplements, you will be taking cod liver oil, Calphonite and a flaxseed drink, which appear in the following daily time schedule.

To prepare flaxseed drink, soak 1 tablespoon of flaxseeds in 1/4 cup hot water for 8 hours (soak your first drink the night before you begin the program). Strain and discard seeds; drink only the liquid.

TIME SCHEDULE

SKIN BRUSH

7:00 am:	cleansing drink (see preceding page)
8:30 am:	supplements and flaxseed drink, 2 tablespoons Calphonite
10:00 am:	cleansing drink
11:30 am:	supplements with tea or diluted juice
1:00 pm:	cleansing drink
2:30 pm:	supplements with tea
4:00 pm:	cleansing drink
5:30 pm:	supplements, flaxseed drink
7:00 pm:	cleansing drink
Bedtime:	immediately before retiring - 2 tablespoons Calphonite, 1 tablespoon Cod Liver Oil. (Bedtime should be no later than 9:30 pm.)

As you can see, your supplements are taken 1-1/2 hours after the cleansing drinks.

The evening of your first day on the program, you will have the first colema at 7:30 pm. Thereafter, you are to have two per day—one at 7:30 am and the other at 7:30 pm. REST 1/2 hour after each colema.

THE COLEMA

The secret of this cleansing program is to take a special kind of enema called a "colema" twice a day, and perhaps even three times. An inexpensive piece of equipment called a colema board is used which permits the user to comfortably lie down during the treatments. It has a hole in one end which is placed over the toilet. There is either a 4 or 5 gallon bucket hanging above, over a shower rod, and inside the bucket is a tube which allows water to pass down the rubber tubing through a small plastic tube, which is inserted in the rectum. The plastic tube is smaller than your little finger, and we find that toxic material goes right by it and elimination can take place without having to remove the tube. So the water goes in and the toxic waste material comes out and into the toilet.

This program involves taking two colemas a day. I first thought this would perhaps weaken the bowel; but I found that as the water went into the bowel, elimination was easier and a better tone developed in the bowel. It's not a matter of how harshly you let water into the bowel, how ballooned you make the bowel or even how much you can hold. You eliminate as you need to, and that is what develops a bowel wall.

The colema board and associated parts represent a major advance for those interested in getting involved in their own healing process. Not only does it make a colon treatment possible at home, but it also makes for easier planning of one's routine, time savings and puts you in control of the process. This equipment is lightweight and inexpensive, easily stored and can travel with you. Cutting the board in half and hinging it will allow you to pack it into a handy travel bag acceptable to most transportation systems.

INSTRUCTIONS FOR TAKING A COLEMA

The colema board has been designed to provide a safe and easy way to take a high enema. Once you are in the correct position, it is possible to relax and virtually enjoy the rest of the procedure. Both hands are free so you may massage the abdomen and colon. For best results, massaging is most important.

Place body-temperature water in a four or five gallon plastic bucket; do not fill completely. The pail of water may hang on a hook, shower rod or be placed on a sink top or box. Make sure that your bucket is sturdy enough to hold 5 gallons of water and that your hanging point is strong enough to hold the full bucket. There should be approximately four feet between the colema board and the bottom of the pail. Add the mixture you are using (coffee and vinegar, clay water or garlic) into the water.

Place the working end of the colema board over the toilet. The top of the board, where the head rests, may be placed on a chair or the side of the tub for convenience. To prevent splashing of expelled fecal matter, place the lid for the splash board over the end area of the colema board. Check to make sure the water can run freely through the tube which goes to the rectum.

Place a folded towel or foam pad on the board so that it will be comfortable to lie on. Before inserting the colema tip into the tube on the board, rinse well. Apply a small amount of lubricant on the rectal tube so colema tip will be easily inserted, being careful not to clog the holes. Position your body on colema board in order to easily insert the colema tip into the rectum. Slide body down until the buttocks touch the wooden edges of the support.

Open clamp to allow the solution to flow into the colon. You do not have to remove the rectal tip in order to evacuate. The fecal matter will bypass the tip, allowing normal bowel action. The colema board encourages normal peristalsis without producing bowel distension. Begin abdomen massage. Start massaging upward on your left side. If you find any tender or sore areas, continue to massage until the tenderness is gone. Continue up to the ribs on the left, then across the abdomen and down the right side. This brings the solution to the ascending colon. When cramping or the desire to evacuate occurs, close off the water clamp (in-flow) and simply relieve the bowel. The small, pencil-like tip will allow free elimination without being removed.

Continue this procedure until you have eliminated the bulk of fecal mass or until you have exhausted the water contents in the bucket. This will normally take about 30 minutes. Be sure to clamp off tube before all the water is used, iin order to maintain the siphon action in the hose.

Upon completion of the colema, clean the board and tubes with a germicidal solution. When removing the tip for cleaning, be sure to replace the piece of 1/4-inch rubber tubing that holds the tip on the adjustable holder of the rectal tube. It is suggested that the tip be immersed in a germicidal solution and stored until the next colema.

SIPHONING THE HOSE

To start the water flow in the hose you must siphon it. This is accomplished by putting the end that goes in the bucket under the faucet. Run water through it, past the u-tube, then hold it up in the air so the water can run down the long part of the hose. Once it has run down, close the clamp, then start it in the same way you did before and your siphon will be working. The idea is that when water is pulled down the long part of the hose it will naturally draw the water up the hose from the bucket and around the u-tube.

To keep the siphon flow, always clamp off the hose before the bucket has run dry. This way you will retain your suction without having to resiphon. If the bucket does run dry, you must repeat the starting procedure.

Another way to drain the bucket is to attach a small plastic fitting into a hole at the base of the bucket. Attach the neoprene hose to this fitting and the other end to the colema board.

ADDITIONS TO THE COLEMA WATER SOLUTION

There are a few additives I might mention to use in the colema water. First of all, you can add a pint of coffee. Coffee helps bring down bile from the liver and stimulates the bowel wall to throw out the toxic material faster. You can also add clay water, which I believe has a great effect on the mucus membrane, loosening it and releasing it faster. Of course, this procedure is repeated two times a day for the seven-day period. After the week, the Maintenance Program is followed for seven weeks. It is recommended that you follow this with another cleansing program. I feel this is the Ultimate Cleansing Program, a process which completely and thoroughly removes the toxic material from the bowel.

ADDITIONAL CONSIDERATIONS

The Ultimate Tissue Cleansing System is very good at overcoming pain. Pain of all kinds from any part of the body, such as in arthritis, headaches, etc.

In overcoming serious degenerative disease, it is recommended that the treatment be ongoing and constantly applied for possibly one year and perhaps longer.

It should be understood that this treatment cannot be considered a "cure all," but rather is an important step for leading the body to detoxification and cleansing.

Treatment must be given according to the patient's responsiveness—watch for reactions closely.

Three days may be all a patient can endure to begin with, especially with the elderly and very weak.

One day may be all that can be safely administered if the patient drops in energy level severely. Please remember that reactions can set in quickly and must be attended to at once.

This is the most powerful detoxifying program I know of. Approach it with respect. We are unleashing potent healing powers that may be overwhelming to the uninitiated.

COLEMA BOARD DESIGN

The following photographs illustrate the colema board design, layout and use. It is an essential component to the success of the Ultimate Cleansing Program. **Note:** The colema boards seen in this book are patended devices; exact replication will result in an infringement of patent rights and therefore this must be avoided. For those who wish to purchase a board ready-made, or are seeking component parts, the following companies are listed: Colema Boards, Inc., Bon Roy Enterprises, Ultimate Colonics, Jennings Home Colonic Boards, V.E. Irons, Inc., and in Canada, Take Care Health Products. (See Bibliography for addresses.)

I feel that all the boards pictured below do the same job. They are made by the different companies and you can pick one you like. We have used Colema Boards, Inc., since first instituting this program.

1. Be sure the 5-gallon bucket is at least 4 feet above the patient and in a stable and safe position.

2. The bucket can be hung if the weight can be supported properly.

3. Start the siphon by filling the tube with water and immersing it in a full bucket of colema water.

4. The board measures 45-1/2 inches by 15-1/2 inches, and is a patented device.

5. The head end of the board must be supported by using the bath tub, stool or chair.

6. Detail of working end of colema board showing inlet tube.

7. The colema rectal tip is approximately 8 inches long and 1/4 inches in diameter.

8. Lubricate the tip before using with K-Y Jelly.

9. Inserting the tip into the flexible tube.

10. Tip in place.

11. Splash lid in place.

12. Ready for use.

13. Working end detail showing relative size and position of parts.

14. Long view of board in place.

15. Placing the splash lid over exit end and showing more detail.

16. Make yourself comfortable for 1/2 to 3/4 hour.

17. It's really very simple and not complicated at all!

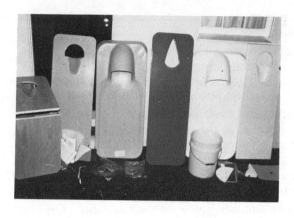

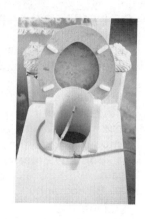

Colema boards in various positions, and the use of the board: placement in small rooms, mobile homes, etc., folding boards for traveling — carried in suitcases.

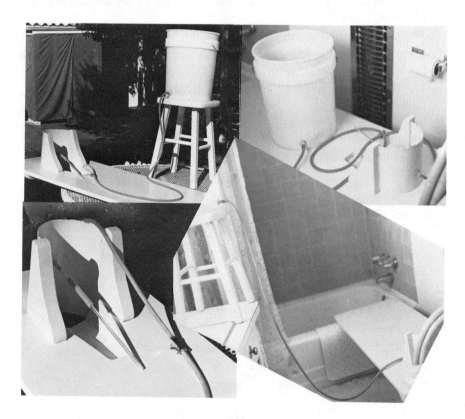

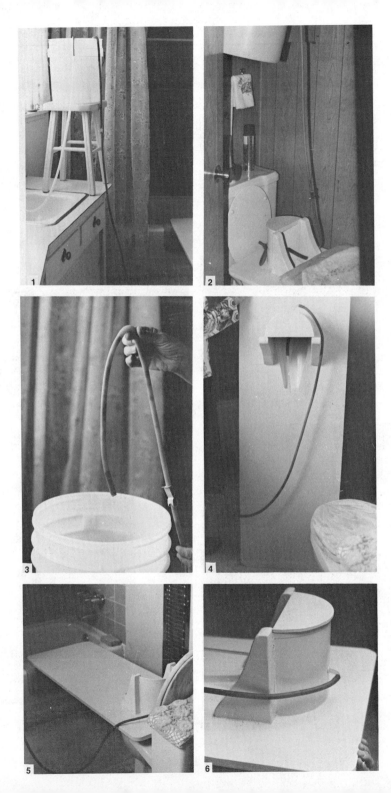

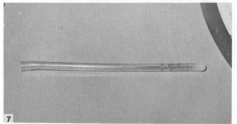

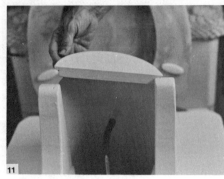

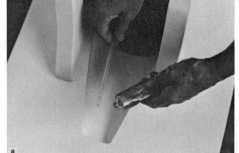

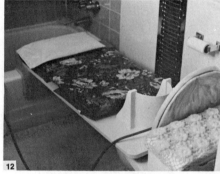

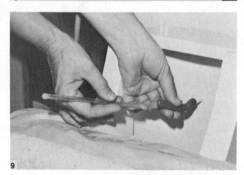

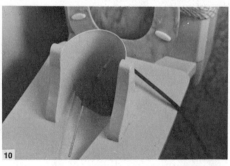

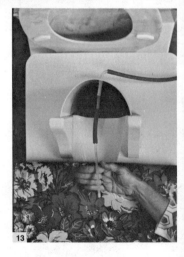

117

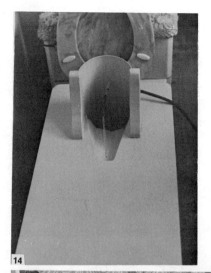

14

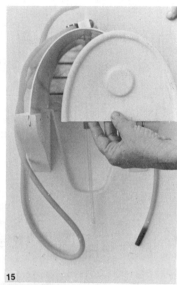

15

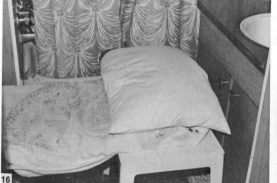

16

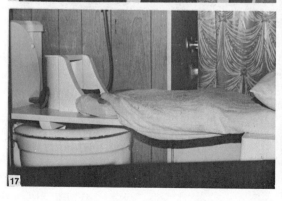

17

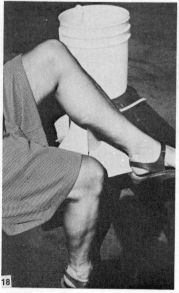

18

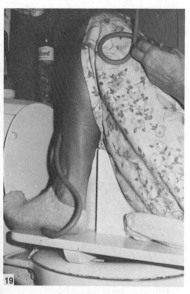

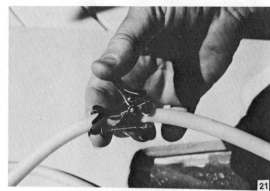

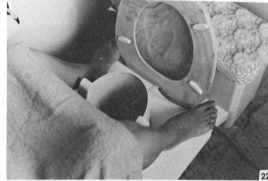

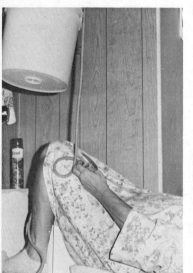

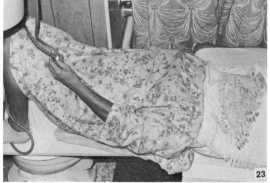

18. Seat yourself down and pull your legs up, moving the buttocks forward. Do **not** insert tip more than 3 inches in rectum.

19. Buttocks are to come in contacts with the stops.

20. Operate the clamp controls with a free hand, releasing the water solution.

21. Simple clamp controls water flow; you do it yourself, so you have complete control.

22. Ready to go.

23. Relax and rest during the treatment.

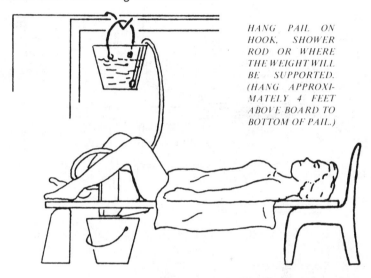

HANG PAIL ON HOOK, SHOWER ROD OR WHERE THE WEIGHT WILL BE SUPPORTED. (HANG APPROXIMATELY 4 FEET ABOVE BOARD TO BOTTOM OF PAIL.)

USE GREAT CAUTION

Insert plastic rectal tip no more than 3 inches past anus, because the distance between the anus and the bend in the bowel where the sigmoid flexure joins the rectum is only about 5 inches in most persons and less in some. Pressing the plastic tip in too far could result in irritation to the bowel wall.

Colema pail may hang on hook, shower rod or set on sink top or box. Colema board may have the "working end" placed over a 5-gallon pail with head end on chair, or the entire board may be placed on bathtub with 5-gallon pail under "working end." You can also place it over the toilet.

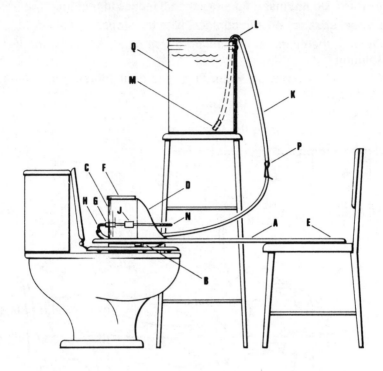

A Colema board
B Valley or excrement drain
C Splash board
D Buttock support
E Head area of board
F Lid for splash board
G Plastic connector (passes through splash board)
H "L" shaped tube
J Latex surgical tubing (short, 3")
K Latex surgical tubing (long)
L Latex-filled "U" tubing (hooks over edge of bucket)
M Metal tip (to keep end of tube close to bottom of bucket)
N Colon tip
P Clamp (to control water flow)
Q Pail (not included)

COLEMA PREPARATION

Morning Colema

Add 1 pint of coffee and 2 tablespoons apple cider vinegar to a little less than 5 gallons of water. (To prepare coffee, allow 2 tablespoons of coffee to 1 pint of water; bring to a rolling boil; let stand 15 minutes before using. You may want to make a 2-day supply of coffee each time). Massage abdomen in rolling motion or use vibrator on colon, working from left side up to transverse colon, across abdomen left to right, down ascending colon the right side.

Evening Colema

Add 1/2 to 1 cup of clay water to 5 gallons of water. Repeat massage or use vibrator. **DO NOT MIX COFFEE AND CLAY WATER BECAUSE THEY COUNTERACT ONE ANOTHER.**

If you think you may have worms, you can substitute garlic enemas for the clay water on the third and fourth days of the program. (Even if you do not have worms, this is a good bowel cleanser). To prepare, place four unpeeled garlic cloves (clean) in a blender with one cup of water; liquefy, strain liquid and add to the colema water; take the colema as usual. Molasses colemas are also good; add 2 tablespoons molasses to the colema water. No other ingredient is added.

During the 7-day program, you may wish to have massages, foot reflexology or epsom salt baths; all are good.

Optional After Colemas

You may use rectal implants. All implants are placed in a baby enema syringe and squeezed into the rectum. For colitis or bleeding, use 1 cup of flaxseed tea and 2 tablespoons of liquid chlorophyll or use 3 to 5 crushed Green Life tablets, and insert as much liquid as can be held. To assist elimination, add 1 heaping tablespoon of Green Life powder, 1/3 cup clay water and add distilled water to thin the mixture enough to let it flow freely through the syringe.

After the 7-day program, drink acidophilus culture for one month. Use 1 cup morning and night; this should follow each 7-day program. (Recommended: Continental, Kovac brands or Eugalan Topfer Forte).

Get specific instructions from your doctor with regard to future supplements.

It is advised to go through the 7-day program again after 7 weeks.

CONCLUDING THE TISSUE CLEANSING TREATMENT

In order to reintroduce the bowel to regular meals, it is suggested that the following program be implemented. This mini diet will prepare the digestive organs for normal functioning and make the transition from the cleansing treatment to regular meals very smooth.

FIRST DAY:

Breakfast: Shredded carrots, slightly wilted.
Lunch: Large salad; yogurt or cottage cheese or nut milk drink.
Dinner: Large salad; one steamed vegetable.

SECOND DAY:

Breakfast: Fresh fruit or dried fruit, revived; cereal or soft-boiled egg.
Lunch: Large salad; one steamed vegetable; yogurt or cottage cheese or nut milk drink.
Dinner: Large salad; one steamed vegetable; a protein.
Eat lightly, slowly and chew well. Teas and juices are allowed between meals, as desired.

THIRD DAY:

Start regular diet.

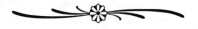

MAINTENANCE PROGRAM
AND ONGOING
REJUVENATION SCHEDULE

This maintenance program is designed to be followed after the 7-Day Cleansing Program. You will stay on this maintenance program for seven (7) weeks, then go back on the 7-Day Cleansing Program, then back again on the maintenance program, which you will now continue for six to eight months.

SCHEDULE

1. **7-Day Cleansing Program**
2. **Maintenance Program - 7 weeks**
3. **7-Day Cleansing Program again**
4. **Maintenance Program—6 to 8 months**

INSTRUCTIONS FOR THE MAINTENANCE PROGRAM

Daily	Skin brush, 3-5 minutes.
CLEANSING DRINK	Twice a day, morning and night.
Part One:	2 oz apple juice 8 oz water 1 tablespoon clay water 1 teaspoon intestinal cleanser SHAKE WELL AND DRINK.
Part Two:	10 oz water 1 tablespoon apple cider vinegar 1 teaspoon honey
SUPPLEMENTS	Three times a day, with meals:
Green Life	Six
Wheat Germ Oil	One
Vitamin C	100 mg two times a day
Niacin	50 mg two times a day
Pancreatin	Two
Beet Tablets	One
Dulse Tablets	One
Calphonite	Two times a day, 1 tablespoon, morning and night.
Cod Liver Oil	Once daily, 1 tablespoon at night.
COLEMA	ONE daily. You may alternate with the following two: Coffee and Vinegar: 1 cup of coffee per colema with 2 tablespoons vinegar; or Clay Water—1/2 to 1 cup per 5 gallon water. (If you feel as if you need more than one colema a day during this maintenance, it is alright to have another. If you miss a colema during the 6-8 month period, it is alright too.)
REST	Lots of rest during the day. To bed by 9 or 9:30 pm.

POST COLEMA SUPPLEMENTS AND MAINTENANCE FOODS

Here is a list of supplements that will greatly aid in the body rebuilding itself after the tissue cleansing treatment has been completed. Zinc, vitamin E (800 IU) daily, vitamin C (up to 10,000 mg daily), vitamin A (50,000 IU daily—not artificial, Norwegian fish liver oil is best), Brewer's Yeast, Blackstrap Molasses (unsulfured), Lecithin capsules (2 to 4 daily).

Vitamin A is especially good in all bowel disturbances, ulcerations, colitis and getting rid of infections. Combined with vitamin F, the two are the greatest supplements for all mucus linings.

Use brewer's yeast to obtain a supplementation of the B vitamins.

For a little extra energy use a teaspoonful of honey in a glass of water.

A good way to start the day is with two tablespoons of natural apple cider vinegar to one glass of warm water every morning before breakfast. It is also good for those who are trying to reduce weight because it is a fat reducer. Also it is very high in potassium which supports the heart, cleans up bladder infections and aids in changing the bowel flora toward the friendly side.

Another good idea is to use one teaspoon of liquid chlorophyll in a glass of water before breakfast.

Here is a list of the most powerful building foods. Sunflower seed butter, sesame seed butter, almond butter, raw goat's cheese, cheese that breaks (aged), baked yams, whole brown rice, yellow cornmeal, rye, millet, sardines, tofu, avocado, cottage cheese, clabber milk, eggs, beans and legumes.

Here are the most cleansing and infection-fighting foods. Green peppers, tomatoes, fresh peas, watercress, all squashes, all kinds of berries, melons, greens (parsley especially), vegetable juices and fruit juices, turnips (juice of) and raw foods.

After the treatment, you can use sauerkraut (saltless preferred) for a natural laxative. Use it also for any signs of constipation.

QUESTIONS AND ANSWERS ABOUT THE COLEMA TREATMENT

QUESTION   For what particular reason is a flaxseed enema taken?

ANSWER   It can be taken at any time, but in particular if you have a bleeding bowel, because flaxseed is very healing. Also for a bleeding bowel, add a couple of teaspoons of liquid chlorophyll to the flaxseed enema. This will help any inflammation of the bowel.

QUESTION   How many dairy products should we have?

ANSWER   Too many dairy products produce mucus, catarrh and bronchial troubles. One or two glasses of milk a day will not cause much damage however. There are milk substitutes such as a nut milk drink that will not produce catarrh. You can also get a natural cheese made from raw whole milk.

QUESTION   You told us to have white fish with fins. What particular fish is that?

ANSWER   Sea trout, cod, sole, salmon, halibut—any fish with scales and fins. Frozen fish can be used, but fresh is preferred.

QUESTION   In taking the niacin, I get such a flush and I itch and bleed, but this doesn't happen when I take the time-release niacin.

ANSWER   The program calls for 100 mg of niacin 3 times a day, so you can cut it down to 25 mg 3 times a day. The flush is needed to force the blood into parts of your intestinal tract where there are infections. Just as you get a flush on the outside, you will also get a flush on the inside.

QUESTION   Should we take 1 teaspoon or 1 tablespoon of cod liver oil, and should it be taken with the Calphonite to bypass the liver and go directly to the bloodstream?

ANSWER   Take 1 tablespoon before the Calphonite. Don't worry about bypassing anything. Follow directions explicitly and don't worry about it.

QUESTION	Why is it necessary to take the Calphonite first?
ANSWER	You don't take Calphonite first. Take the cod liver oil first; it seems to sit better without gagging. Take the cod liver oil at night before retiring, so it will travel through the gall bladder and liver without much stirring up.
QUESTION	How do you get off this fast?
ANSWER	First, let it be known that it is not a true fast. A fast means complete abstinence from nutrients. This is a cleansing program and the way to end it is with soft fruits like peaches or soft apricots. Shredded, wilted carrots can be taken and also slightly wilted apples. You should also have a cooked vegetable, carrots or beets. Between meals, you can have celery juice, carrot juice or vegetable broth. The day following, you may have cereal with revived fruits or a banana for breakfast. Shredded carrots, millet cereal and a small salad at lunch. In the evening, you may have another salad and a cooked vegetable. The next day, you can start on my regular diet.
QUESTION	How should I conduct myself during the day while on this elimination?
ANSWER	The more rest you give your body, the better. Take a short walk. Take your colemas and afterward rest at least half an hour. But rest is most important.
QUESTION	What about eating shrimp and crab?
ANSWER	Do not include these in your diet.
QUESTION	Is it alright to have a coffee substitute with no grain?
ANSWER	All coffee substitutes are poor; but if you must use it, try Pero or Sanocaf, both are made in Switzerland.
QUESTION	How long are we on this elimination?
ANSWER	I recommend the 7-day cleansing but the length of time is determined on an individual case basis.

QUESTION	Is it better to use the colema in the morning or evening?
ANSWER	I prefer morning—but do it once a day. After 2-3 months, you can even skip a day if necessary. Take the bulk and clay water twice a day, morning and night.
QUESTION	Should we alternate between the coffee and clay water colema?
ANSWER	Coffee is the best to take every day and just once a day.
QUESTION	What other supplements should be taken?
ANSWER	The supplements stated for this cleansing program should be taken because they are slanted toward cleansing. Supplements for building should be determined by your doctor, according to your particular condition.
QUESTION	Should I take acidophilus bacteria while on the tissue cleansing and colema treatment?
ANSWER	No, but take it afterward. Take it when you return home, perhaps as an implant. You can do it for a month or two after this program.
QUESTION	I'm already exhausted; I feel I could be in bed right now. How will this be over the 7 days?
ANSWER	This is the second day—and you are one of the unusual ones because of your past problems. The more elimination you have, the less energy you will have also. Cleansing requires a lot of rest. We will not take you the full 7 days due to your past history.
QUESTION	I make goat milk cheese; should I drink the whey?
ANSWER	Yes, whey is the greatest thing for the stomach to make hydrochloric acid needed for digestion.
QUESTION	Is it too high in sodium for me?
ANSWER	No, because you won't be taking a large amount.
QUESTION	On this cleansing, if I experience pain or gas, should I take another colema?

ANSWER	Yes; in all cases of pain or intestinal distress, it is best to take another colema and it can be done in succession without any harm.
QUESTION	Can chicken bones be used in the veal broth soup? And should they be raw or can they be from a roasted chicken?
ANSWER	Yes, you can use chicken bones and raw is preferred; although roasted chicken bones can be used also.
QUESTION	Why are we drinking the vinegar/honey mixture?
ANSWER	It helps do some of the work that hydrochloric acid does in the stomach in digesting proteins. It stirs up the acid-alkaline balance in the body to throw off more acids through the urine.
QUESTION	Will an overdose of calcium cause muscle cramps?
ANSWER	Yes, it could.
QUESTION	How do we control calcium?
ANSWER	Good stomach digestion. Iodine controls calcium. Greens, tops of vegetables, also control calcium.
QUESTION	I'm worried about my weight on this cleansing.
ANSWER	Most people on this elimination diet do not lose much, if any, weight. You are not totally fasting, you are having juices and the vitamins and minerals which are all foods.
QUESTION	When should I take the Digestaid tablets?
ANSWER	During your meals.
QUESTION	Will you tell us about implants? What should be used?
ANSWER	Implants are inserted with a baby enema syringe (about 1 cup of liquid) into the rectum at bedtime, and should be held overnight. The best implant is acidophilus culture. Use this for 2-3 months after the cleansing, skip 2-3 months and start using the implant again. We are replacing the friendly bacteria in the bowel using acidophilus culture. Of course, during the day, you can take acidophilus orally. We all have a lack

of the friendly bacteria, but even more so in taking frequent colemas.

Other implants to use are garlic oil in water; flaxseed tea; liquid chlorophyll; crushed Green Life tablets and water. Clay water is a very soothing implant to use occasionally. Aloe vera gel and water can also be used as a healer for the inflamed tissue of the colon. The implants should all be used at body temperature; the rectum will expel cold water quicker.

Some doctors recommend yogurt or buttermilk as implants, these are fine, but when on the colema treatments, I feel the ones I've mentioned above are best. Buttermilk implants can help remove extreme intestinal gas.

Vinegar and water implants can help rid the bowel of acid and germ life. Garlic oil can help eliminate pinworms in children.

QUESTION   Does the bowel become better using colemas, and will the water reach the small intestine?

ANSWER   I believe the large intestine is best cared for through colemas and eventually it becomes stronger. The tone built up will be transferred to the whole bowel. The most difficult to care for is the ascending colon where the toxic material is thrown into the large colon. As you develop bowel tone, better bowel movements are attained and there is less toxic material to deal with, so the tissue becomes better.

QUESTION   Can diverticuli be reversed?

ANSWER   This condition represents a combination of inherited bowel qualities and improper diet/eating habits. It can be corrected with colemas, proper eating and proper exercises, using the slant board.

QUESTION   Why do I feel weak, especially after the colema?

ANSWER   Colemas are a cleansing treatment, and your body is working to remove toxic material. That's why you're weak and that's why it is so important to rest for half an hour after each colema.

QUESTION	Should we continue with the vinegar and honey at mealtime when we go home?
ANSWER	Take the bulk, vinegar and honey twice a day, morning and night, when you go off the fast. This will continue for several months.
QUESTION	I've noticed my heart seems to be pounding; could it be overworking?
ANSWER	It could be that you're working more and you should rest. The pounding could also be caused by gas pressure.
QUESTION	Is it better to crush the tablets we are taking now?
ANSWER	No, just crack them once before swallowing.
QUESTION	What can I do to make my body absorb proteins better?
ANSWER	Emotional strain breaks down this ability more than anything. Then, of course, we have to get sodium back into the stomach wall to help digest protein. Take the more easily digested proteins also.
QUESTION	Clay water seems to constipate me in taking the colema. Coffee seems to work better.
ANSWER	Clay water does have a tendency toward constipation—but it is very soothing to an irritated bowel. It absorbs 90 times its own weight of acid excretions in the bowel, so it is the greatest cleanser available. It attracts material to be eliminated. The coffee enema is a stimulant to most people. You can't be constipated very long on this treatment.
QUESTION	Can I mix coffee with the clay water?
ANSWER	It's best not to mix the two, because they have separate effects. Clay water is quite alkaline and coffee is acid. That's why you use cider vinegar in the coffee enema.
QUESTION	Is it better to take the colema before or after supplements?
ANSWER	Take supplements after the colema.

QUESTION   What is the best time of day to take the colema?

ANSWER   In the morning. If this isn't possible, take it at night, but
             take it once a day.

See chart
p. 154

HERING'S LAW OF CURE

I work with the purest ideas possible, the best foods possible, the
best processes possible, and in working with these ideals, we work with
the reversal process. As you have built up the disease through the acute,
subacute, chronic and degenerative stages, we reverse and correct
these conditions as we go back over our past problems. As you have
built up conditions in the body through foods, pollution, overwork,
enervation, lifestyle, etc., we have to learn our lesson and go back over
them and relive them, so to speak. You can expect all of these problems
to return as you get well. This is best described in my book *DOCTOR-
PATIENT HANDBOOK*. If you truly want to get well, this process must
be followed.

We find that "Hering's Law of Cure" appears in the reversal process
as healing takes place. In this process the body eliminates iatrogenic
symptoms and diseases, those things caused by treatments that were
suppressive in nature and usually involved a drug of some kind.

Latent settlements of any foreign accumulations leave the body
mainly through the bowel as a liquified form of mucus or catarrh.

For example, we had an asthma patient who received much relief
from the tissue cleansing treatment but developed an extreme uterine
abscess which broke shortly after the treatment and discharged the
foulest material possible and continued for a month after.

She lost extreme weight and will not gain until after the discharge
culminates. She needed the assistance of a tissue cleansing treatment
to bring on an elimination. This latent tumor or abscess was
suppressed. Discharge from lungs, bronchials, head, ears and nose for
17 years, and of course, always suppressed it with some form of drug.

I have said so many times—if you suppress or don't allow a
discharge to continue until you are clean inside, you will develop a
growth—and she did just that.

133

INSTRUCTIONS FOR SKIN BRUSHING

I believe skin brushing is one of the finest of all baths. No soap can wash the skin as clean as the new skin you have under the old. You make new skin every 24 hours on the body. The skin will be as clean as the blood is.

Skin brushing removes this top layer. This helps to eliminate uric acid crystals, catarrh and various other acids in the body. The skin should eliminate two pounds of waste acids daily. Keep the skin active. No one can be well wearing clothes unless they brush their skin. It is the greatest method to remove the scurf rim as found in the eye, which denotes an underactive, poorly eliminating skin.

Use a natural bristle brush with a long handle. It is not an expensive brush. **DO NOT USE A NYLON BRISTLE BRUSH.** Use this brush dry, first thing in the morning when you arise before putting clothes on and before any bath. Use it in any direction all over the whole body except the face. You can use a special face brush for the face.

DR. JENSEN'S BALANCED DAILY EATING REGIMEN

Make a habit of applying the following General Diet Regimen to your everyday living. This is a healthy way to live because when followed, you do not have to think of vitamins, mineral elements or calories. I will give you more specific instruction for your troubles after you have made this daily regimen automatic.

The best diet, over a period of a day, is two different fruits, at least four to six vegetables, one protein and one starch, with fruit or vegetable juices between meals. Eat at least two green leafy vegetables a day. The foods you eat daily should be 50-60% raw. Consider this regimen a dietetic law.

RULES OF EATING

1. Do not fry foods or use heated oils.
2. If not entirely comfortable in mind and body from the previous meal time, you should miss the next meal.
3. Do not eat unless you have a keen desire for the plainest food.
4. Do not eat beyond your needs.
5. Be sure to thoroughly masticate your food.
6. Miss meals if in pain, emotionally upset, not hungry, chilled, overheated and during acute illness.

GOOD THOUGHTS, GOOD WORDS, GOOD DEEDS
(The Formula for Healthy Living)

Learn to accept whatever decision is made.

Let the other person make a mistake and learn.

Learn to forgive and forget.

Be thankful and bless people.

Live in harmony—even if it is good for you.

Do not talk about your illness.

Gossip will kill you. Don't let anyone gossip to you either. Gossip that comes through the grapevine is usually sour grapes.

Be by yourself every day for 10 minutes with the thought of how to make yourself a better person. Replace negative thoughts with uplifting, positive thoughts.

Skin brush daily. Use a slant board daily.

Have citrus fruit in sections only, never in juice form.

Have only a limited amount of bread (with a lot of bowel trouble, no bread).

Exercise daily. Keep your spine limber. Develop abdominal muscles. Do sniff breathing.

Grass and sand walk for happy feet.

No smoking, alcoholic drinking, spitting or cussing. Keep away from unclean people.

Bed at sundown, 9 pm at the latest, if you are at all tired, fatigued or unable to do your work with vim and vigor. If you are sick, you must rest more. Sleep out of doors, out of the city, in circulating air. Work out problems in the morning, don't take them to bed with you.

FOOD HEALING LAWS

1. Natural food—50-60% of the food eaten should be raw.
2. Your diet should be 80% alkaline and 20% acid. Look at the acid/alkaline chart in *Vital Foods for Total Health*, page 100.
3. Proportion: 6 vegetables daily, 2 fruits daily, 1 starch daily and 1 protein daily.
4. Variety. Vary sugars, proteins, starches, vegetables and fruits from meal to meal and day to day.
5. Overeating. You can kill yourself with the amount of food you eat.
6. Combinations. Separate starches and proteins. One at lunch and the other at dinner. Have fruits for breakfast and at 3 pm.
7. Cook without water. Cook without high heat. Cook without air touching hot foods.
8. Bake, broil or roast. If you eat meat, have it lean, no fat, no pork. Use unsprayed vegetables if possible and eat them as soon after picked as possible.
9. Use stainless steel, low-heat cooking utensils.

BEFORE BREAKFAST. Upon rising and at least 1/2 hour before breakfast, take any natural, unsweetened fruit juice such as grape, pineapple, prune, fig, apple or black cherry. Liquid chlorophyll can be used, 1 teaspoon in a glass of tepid water.

You can have a broth and lecithin drink if you desire. Take 1 teaspoonful of vegetable broth powder and 1 tablespoon of lecithin granules and dissolve both in a glass of warm water.

Between fruit juice and breakfast, follow this program: Skin brushing, exercising, deep breathing or playing. Shower. Start with warm water and cool off until your breath quickens. Never shower immediately upon rising.

BREAKFAST. Stewed fruit, one starch and health drink or two fruits, one protein and health drink. (Starches and health drinks are listed with the lunch suggestions.) Soaked fruits, such as unsulphured apricots, prunes, figs. Fruit of any kind: melon, grapes, peaches, pears, berries or baked apple, which may be sprinkled with some ground nuts or nut butter. When possible, use fruit in season.

SUGGESTED BREAKFAST MENUS

MONDAY
Reconstituted Dried Apricots
Steel-Cut Oatmeal/Supplements
Oat Straw Tea
Add Eggs, if desired
OR
Sliced Peaches
Cottage Cheese/Supplements
Herb Tea

TUESDAY
Fresh Figs
Cornmeal Cereal/Supplements
Shave Grass Tea
Add Eggs or Nut Butter, if desired
OR
Raw Applesauce and Blackberries
Coddled Egg/Supplements
Herb Tea

WEDNESDAY
Reconstituted Dried Peaches
Millet Cereal/Supplements
Alfamint Tea
Add Eggs, Cheese or Nut Butter, if desired
OR
Sliced Nectarines and Apple
Yogurt/Supplements
Herb Tea

THURSDAY
Prunes or any reconstituted dried fruit
Whole Wheat Cereal/Supplements
Oat Straw Tea
OR
Grapefruit and Kumquats
Poached Egg/Supplements
Herb Tea

FRIDAY
Slices of fresh Pineapple with shredded Coconut
Buckwheat Cereal/Supplements
Peppermint Tea
OR
Baked Apple, Persimmons
Chopped raw Almonds/Acidophilus Milk/Supplements
Herb Tea

SATURDAY
Muesli with Bananas and Dates
Cream - Supplements
Dandelion Coffee or Herb Tea

SUNDAY
Cooked Applesauce with Raisins
Rye Grits/Supplements
Shave Grass Tea
OR
Cantaloupe and Strawberries
Cottage Cheese/Supplements
Herb Tea

PREPARATION HELPS. Reconstituted Dried Fruit: Cover with cold water, bring to boil and leave to stand overnight. Raisins may just have boiling water poured over them. This kills any insects and eggs.

Whole Grain Cereal: To cook properly with as little heat as possible, use a double boiler or thermos-cook.

Supplements: (Add to cereal or fruit). Sunflower seed meal, rice polishings, wheat germ, flaxseed meal (about a teaspoon of each). Even a little dulse may be sprinkled over with some broth powder.

10:30 am. Vegetable broth, vegetable juice or fruit juice.

LUNCH. Raw salad, or as directed, one or two starches, listed, and a health drink. Get salad suggestions from Dr. Jensen's cookbook and food guide, *Vital Foods for Total Health.*

NOTE: If following a strict regimen, use only one of the first seven starches daily. Vary the starch from day to day.

RAW SALAD VEGETABLE SUGGESTIONS. Tomatoes (citrus), lettuce (green leafy type only such as romaine), celery, cucumber, beansprouts, green peppers, avocado, parsley, watercress, endive, onion (s) and cabbage (s). (s—denotes sulphur foods.)

STARCHES. Yellow cornmeal, baked potato, baked banana (or at least dead ripe), barley (a winter food), steamed brown rice or wild rice, millet (as a cereal), banana or hubbard squash, steel-cut oatmeal, whole wheat cereal, Dr. Jackson's meal, whole grain Roman Meal, shredded wheat bread (whole wheat, rye, soybean, cornbread, bran muffins, Rye Krisp).

DRINK SUGGESTIONS. Vegetable broth, soup, coffee substitute, buttermilk, raw milk, oat straw tea, alfamint tea, huckleberry tea, papaya tea or any health drink.

SUGGESTED LUNCH MENUS

MONDAY
Vegetable Salad
Baby Lima Beans, Baked Potato
Spearmint Tea

TUESDAY
Vegetable Salad with Health Mayonnaise
Steamed Asparagus
Very ripe Bananas or Steamed Unpolished Rice
Vegetable Broth or Herb Tea

WEDNESDAY
Raw Salad Plate w/Sour Cream dressing
Cooked Green Beans and/or Baked Hubbard Squash
Cornbread
Sassafras Tea

THURSDAY
Salad w/French Dressing
Baked Zucchini and Okra
Corn on the Cob
Rye Krisp
Buttermilk or Herb Tea

FRIDAY
Salad
Baked Green Pepper stuffed with Eggplant & Tomatoes
Baked Potato and/or Bran Muffin
Carrot Soup or Herb Tea

SATURDAY
Salad
Steamed Turnips and Turnip Greens
Baked Yam
Catnip Tea

SUNDAY
Salad w/Lemon & Olive Oil Dressing
Steamed Whole Barley
Cream of Celery Soup
Steamed Chard
Herb Tea

SALAD VEGETABLES. Use plenty of greens. Choose 4 or 5 vegetables from the following: leaf lettuce, watercress, spinach, beet leaves, parsley, alfalfa sprouts, cabbage, young chard, herbs, any green leaves, cucumbers, beansprouts, onions, green peppers, pimientos, carrots, turnips, zucchini, asparagus, celery, okra, radishes, etc.

Vital Foods for Total Health, Nature's Own Cookbook by Bernard Jensen, DC, is a complete food guide. Tables for vitamin and mineral guidance, acid and alkaline tables—with complete instructions for perfect combinations to assure you a correct daily balance, designed to get you well and keep you well. This book shows how to cook, prepare and serve foods healthfully.

3:00 pm: Health cocktail, juice or fruit.

PHOTOGRAPHIC DOCUMENTARY

On the following pages you will observe the very unusual results we have obtained from the Ultimate Tissue Cleansing Program. Please note that these specimens are not all from the same body, but represent the flushings from several individuals.

If a photograph was ever worth a thousand words, surely these are, for they speak for themselves. I have not experienced any other method that can consistently and as thoroughly match this one in results. This is truly a major step forward in the battle to overcome toxemia and autointoxication.

On the first three pages you will see the results of the 7-Day Cleansing Program as it reversed a stubborn case of ulcerated feet and ankles. For more details, please refer to page 159, Chapter 9, Patient 1 in our case histories.

On all three pages, the first photo was taken on Day 1 of the treatment; the second photo was taken on Day 4; and the third photo was taken on Day 7 of the cleansing program. The results are remarkable.

On the following pages, you will witness the shocking effluence as it was gathered from the colema flushing. Who would guess that such things could accumulate inside the human body? Could this substance be the source of disease, illness and poor health?

This accumulated material ranged from jelly-like to hard as truck tire rubber; clear to black as tar; fresh to morbidly old; fragments to 3- and 4-foot long ropes, and all with the odor that only speaks of very rotten things.

Notice the mucus lining taking the shape of the bowel, complete with haustrations, striations, strictures and diverticula. This is truly an amazing phenomenon. Please note that these specimens are not all from the same body, but represent the flushings from several individuals.

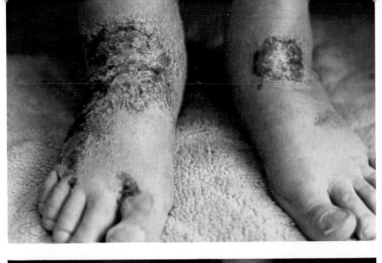

DAY 1

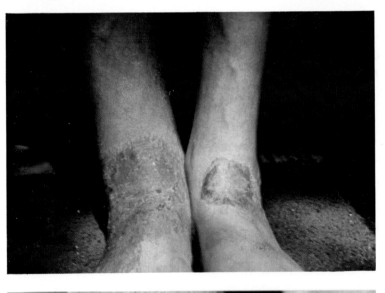

DAY 4

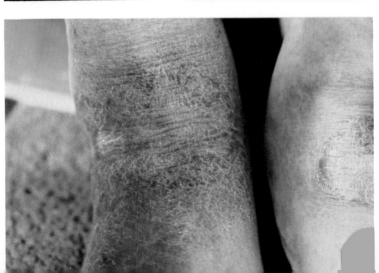

DAY 7

142

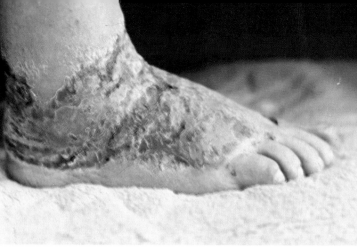

DAY 1

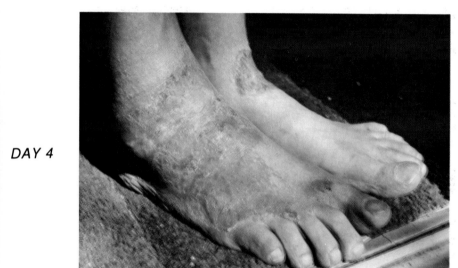

DAY 4

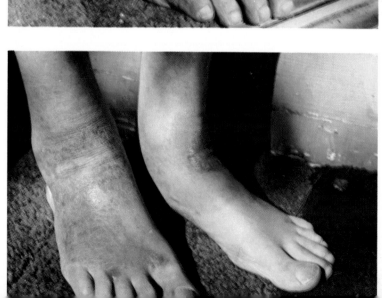

DAY 7

143

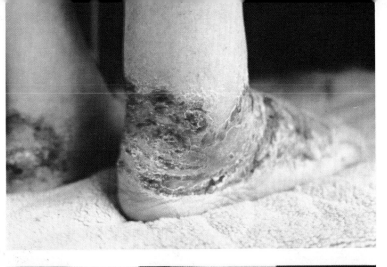

DAY 1

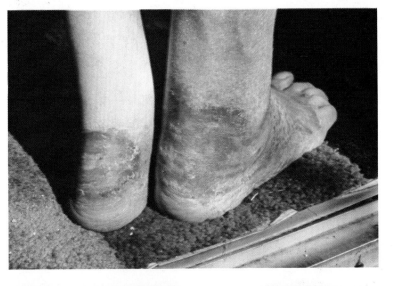

DAY 4

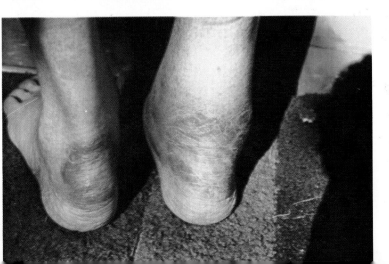

DAY 7

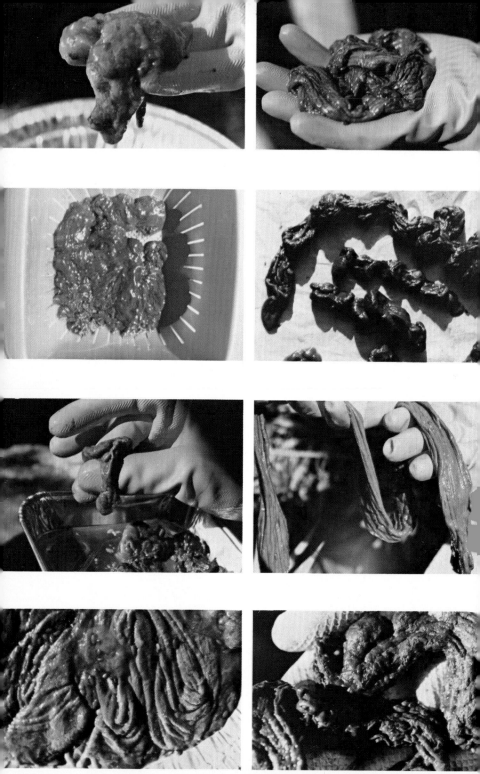

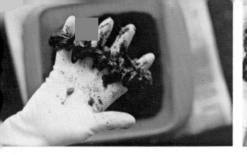

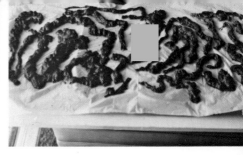

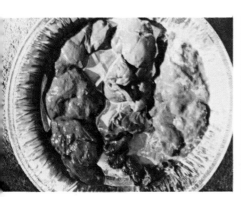

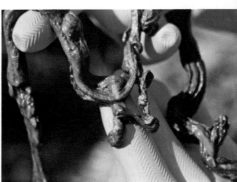

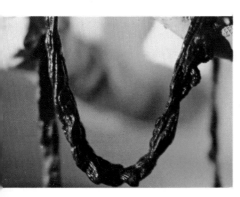

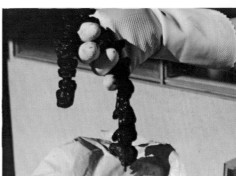

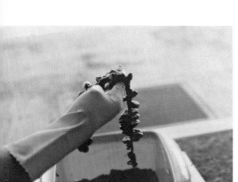

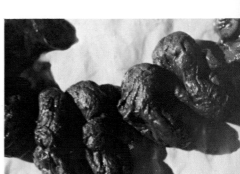

146

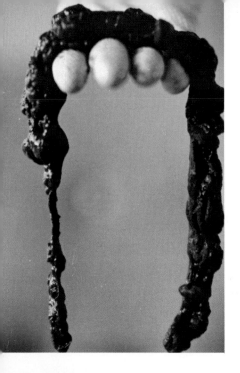

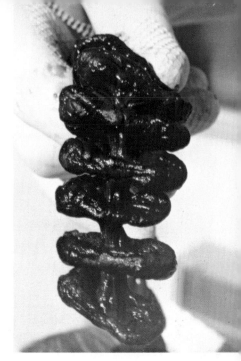

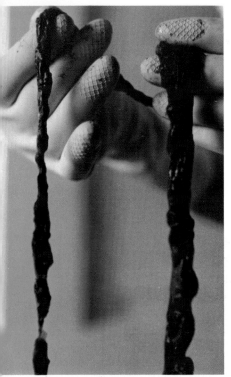

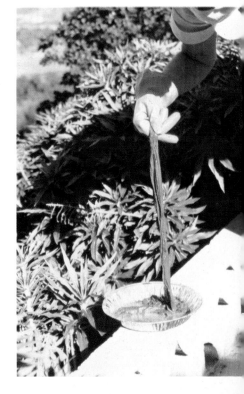

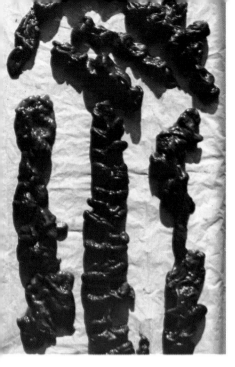

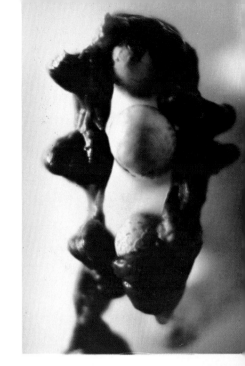

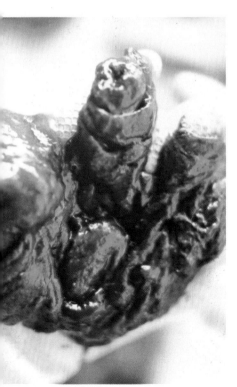

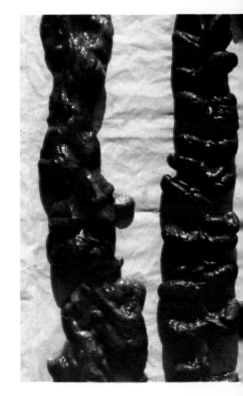

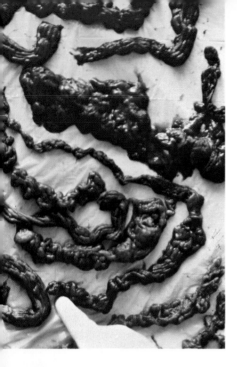
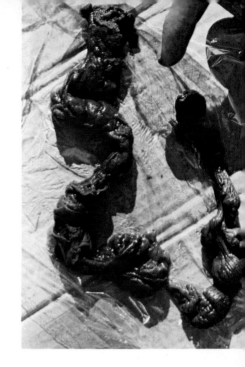
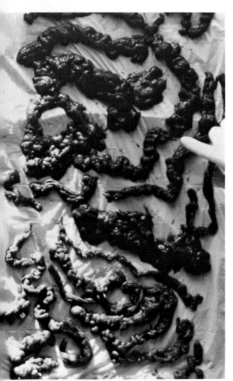
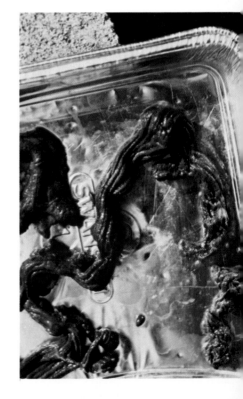

149

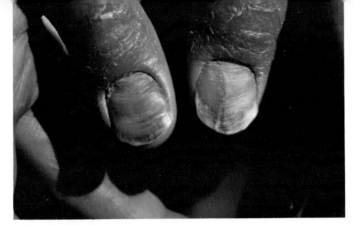

PAINFUL PSORIASIS IN ACUTE STAGE

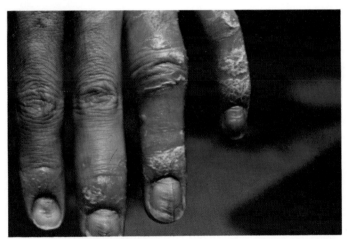

SYMPTOMS RETREAT FOLLOWING TISSUE CLEANSING TREATMENT

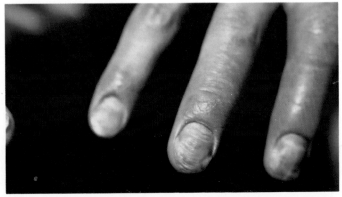

HEALING AND REJUVENATION FOLLOWING DETOXIFICATION 150

Hering's law of cure is clearly illustrated in the following photographs. Here we can see the results of the tissue cleansing treatment as it is combined with good nutritional support. This insulin-dependent diabetic was able to maintain a lower-level blood sugar for the extent of the tissue toxin elimination diet with much less insulin. This patient has had psoriasis for the last 7 years, diabetes for the last 4 years and arthritis for the last 2 years. As you can see, the psoriasis is leaving, as are all the other symptoms. The most recent afflictions are leaving more quickly while the older ones are retreating more slowly, as in the "reverse order."

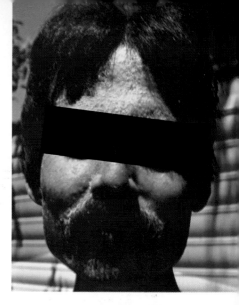

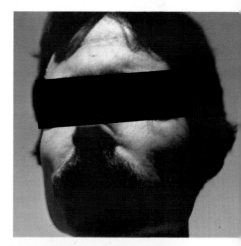

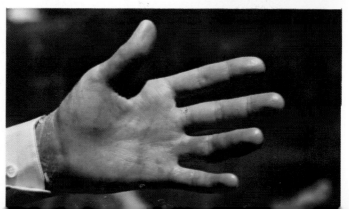

DINNER. Raw salad, two cooked vegetables, one protein and a broth or health drink if desired. Cooked vegetables: peas, artichokes, carrots, beets, turnips, spinach, beet tops, string beans, swiss chard, eggplant, zucchini, summer squash, broccoli (s), cauliflower (s), cabbage (s), sprouts (s), onions (s) or any vegetable other than potatoes. (s— denotes sulfur foods.)

DRINKS. Vegetable broth, soup or health beverage.

PROTEINS

Once a Week: Fish—use white fish, such as sole, halibut, trout or sea trout. Vegetarians: Use soybeans, lima beans, cottage cheese, sunflower seeds and other seeds, also seed butters, nut butters, nut milk drinks, eggs.

Twice a Week: Cottage cheese or any cheese that breaks.

Three times a Week: Meat—use only lean meat; never use pork, fats or cured meats. Vegetarians: Use meat substitutes or vegetarian proteins.

Once a Week: Egg omelet.

If you have a protein at dinner, health dessert is allowed, but not recommended. Never eat protein and starches together. (Notice how they are separated.)

You may exchange your noon meal for the evening meal, but follow the same regimen. It takes exercise to handle raw food, and we generally get more after our noon meal. That is why a raw salad is advised at noon. If you eat sandwiches, have vegetables at the same time.

SUGGESTED DINNER MENUS

MONDAY
Salad
Diced Celery and Carrots
Steamed Spinach
Puffy Omelet
Vegetable Broth

TUESDAY
Salad
Cooked Beet Tops
Steak, broiled or Ground Beef Patties
Cauliflower
Comfrey Tea

WEDNESDAY
Cottage Cheese
Cheese Sticks
Apples, Peaches, Grapes, Nuts
Apple Concentrate Cocktail

THURSDAY
Salad
Steamed Chard
Baked Eggplant
Grilled Liver and Onions
Persimmon Whip (optional)
Alfamint Tea

FRIDAY
Salad w/Yogurt & Lemon Dressing
Steamed Mixed Greens
Beets
Steamed Fish w/Lemon Wedge
Leek Soup

SATURDAY
Salad
Cooked String Beans
Baked Summer Squash
Carrot and Cheese Loaf
Cream of Lentil Soup
Fresh Peach Jell-O w/Almond Nut Cream

SUNDAY
Salad
Diced Carrots and Peas, steamed
Tomato Aspic
Roast Leg of Lamb
Mint Sauce

PATHWAYS TO HEALTH AND DISEASE OBSERVED IN THE IRIS OF THE EYE

ACCORDING TO HERING'S LAW OF CURE: "All cure starts from within out, from the head down and in the reverse order as the symptoms have appeared."

This chart illustrates the correlation between the natural light of the iris and good health versus the darkness of the iris in proportion to the degree of degeneration in the body.

BY BERNARD JENSEN, DC, ND

INDICATION IN IRIS	• WHITE •	• LIGHT GRAY •	• DARK GRAY •	• BLACK •
STAGE	ACUTE	SUBACUTE	CHRONIC	DEGENERATIVE
ASSOCIATED SIGNS	ELEVATED	JUST BELOW SURFACE	WELL BELOW SURFACE	COMPLETELY RECESSED
SYMPTOMS IN BODY	Inflammation, Pain, Sensitivity, Fever, Discharge, High Activity	Toxic, Absorption, Low Metabolism, Weak Condition, Less Pain	Low Metabolic Activity, Toxic buildup, Lack of Vitality	No Sensation, Circulation, Tissue Decay
CATARRH-ACID LEVEL (TOXIC ACCUMULATION)	Poor living habits contribute to the infiltration of catarrhal buildup and the beginning of toxic settlements			Limit of toxic settlement body can tolerate, breakdown of life-giving activity. Vital force at lowest ebb.

DEGENERATIVE PROCESSES: ARTHRITIS, EMPHYSEMA, MALIGNANCY

TISSUE INTEGRITY OR HEALTH LEVEL — HIGH ... LOW

FACTORS THAT UNDERMINE HEALTH & VITALITY:

HEREDITARY FACTORS: Diseases such as Syphilis, Diabetes etc. Alcoholism, Chemical Shortages, Drug Accumulations, B.C. pills, Thalidomide, Tranquilizers etc. X-rays.

CHILDHOOD FACTORS: Accidents. Contagious diseases. Catarrhal accumulations. Poor diet. Pesticides. Sprays. Drugs. Coal tars. Tobacco. Caffeine. Food additives. Weather and Climate conditions. Poor Elimination (Bowel, Lungs, Kidneys, Skin, Lymph.) Nerve depletion. Anemia. Oxygen starvation.

A healing crisis develops on the path at approximately the same point as the original ailment.

Healing Crisis and Reversal Process as shown in the color of the iris.

(WHERE ARE YOU ALONG THIS PATH?)

WE DON'T CATCH DISEASES, WE CREATE THEM BY BREAKING DOWN THE NATURAL DEFENSES ACCORDING TO THE WAY WE EAT, DRINK, THINK AND LIVE.

Suppression: Coal tar drugs, nostrums, aspirin, etc.

COLDS Fatigue, enervation are first to appear (get rid of cold feet)

COUGHS Next to appear

BRONCHITIS

ALLERGIES Eyes change color

FLU

SINUS Discharges from nose, eyes, vagina Boils

HAY FEVER

Suppression: Sprays, vapors, synthetic chemicals

PNEUMONIA

ASTHMA

Healing: Catarrhal eliminations, healing crisis

Healing Catarrhal elimination

HEALING PROCESS PATH

ARTHRITIS PATH

MALIGNANCY PATH

Follows the reversal path and retraces over all past illnesses

Healing: Tissue cleaning, toxic elimination, correct diet

Suppression: Cortisone, chemotherapy, radiation, heavy drugs.

Suppression: Penicillin, antibiotics, sulfa drugs, tranquilizers

MALIGNANCY TUMORS, ARTHRITIS, GANGRENE, EMPHYSEMA, HARDENING OF ARTERIES

TOWARD ILLNESS AND DISEASE

TOWARD HEALING/REJUVENATION

(BIRTH) 2 Years | 11 Years | 28 Years | Any age (DEATH)

COPYRIGHT 1981 DR. BERNARD JENSEN RTE 1 BOX 52 ESCONDIDO CA 92025

CHART TO IRIDOLOGY

RIGHT IRIS   LEFT IRIS

IRIDOLOGY CHART developed by Dr. Bernard Jensen D.C.

(1) FROM THE INSIDE OUT
(2) FROM THE HEAD DOWN
(3) IN THE REVERSE ORDER

FIRST TO HEAL
SECOND TO HEAL
THIRD TO HEAL
FOURTH TO HEAL

THE FUNDAMENTALS FOR STARTING THE REVERSAL PATH TO A HIGHER HEALTH LEVEL

Dis-ease cannot be cured in anyone who practices degenerative lifestyle habits. There is no one specific cause that produces any one specific dis-ease nor is there any one treatment that will correct any one dis-ease.

True healing is a holistic being composed of body, mind and soul. Treatments should be nonivasive, nontoxic, wholistically oriented — such as nutritional, homeopathic, naturopathic, osteopathic, chiropractic, massage, structural exercise, reflexive, hydrotherapic, herbal, physiotherapeutic, color, etc.), geographic, climatic, spiritual, philosophical, etc. These treatments are designed to promote the retracing process to attain higher health levels.

We cannot re-establish balance and equilibrium, to develop light in dark places. This is the path of Hering's Law of Cure. When the body is treated properly, we come out of degeneracy (darkness) to a lighter eye and good health. Iridology leads the way in demonstrating this principle.

Four factors to regain and maintain good health: Nerve supply (mechanical and chemical), Blood supply (cleansing and building), Circulation and Overcoming Enervation.

What prevents a dis-ease will cure a dis-ease. All chronic and degenerative diseases follow the same path of enervation and chemical depletion along with suppression of vital nerve force. All healing starts with the elimination of toxic wastes and removing the darkness found in the iris. True healing is a cleansing and building process. Cure is an ideal that we must constantly strive for. Without ideals we become lost. Cure is premature only when it is permanent. Always welcome a catarrhal discharge instead of ridding the body of poisons. Decide which way you want to go—suppression or elimination. It all depends upon the path you take. Hippocrates. Give me a fever and I'll cure any disease. Hering's philosophy of cure. Give me a fever and I'll cure any disease. Nature cures. Nature cures, but she must be given the opportunity. For an in-depth description of the reversal and healing crisis process, refer to Doctor-Patient Handbook by Dr. Bernard Jensen.

This chart illustrates Hering's law of cure by showing the paths that lead to disease and revitalization, as they are one and the same. This concept is vitally important to the understanding of the "reversal process" and the amazing phenomena of the healing body as it responds to natural, pure and whole remedies. Full color chart measuring 11 by 17 inches is available from the publisher, see last page for address.

THE IMMUNE SYSTEM

The immune system is made up of a system of specialized tissues, cells and antibodies, in addition to that aspect of immunity that we think of as represented by healthy, chemically-balanced organs, glands and tissues in a body with active, clean elimination channels.

External to the body, the skin is our first line of defense against toxins, germlife and viruses. Tears in the eyes and skin perspiration have bacteriocidal properties. Internally, mucous membranes lining the nose, throat and lungs prevent most unwanted microbes from entering the body. Sticky mucus captures the great majority of germs and viruses, which are ejected when the mucus is eliminated. Most germlife taken in food is destroyed by hydrochloric acid in the stomach. Bacteria and viruses that manage to enter the bloodstream or lymph are unable to get through most healthy cellular membranes, and they face almost certain destruction by other parts of the immune system.

The four elimination channels (skin, lungs and bronchials, kidneys, bowel) play an important part in immunity by ridding the body of food wastes and metabolic wastes that would otherwise support the growth and multiplication of harmful germs and viruses. The liver detoxifies the blood as a "backup system" for the elimination channels.

The immune system, strictly speaking, is made up of the lymphatic system, including the spleen, tonsils and appendix and some breast tissue, but also the thymus gland, the Kupfer cells of the liver, and Peyer's patches in the small intestine. The lymph system produces several types of specialized cells capable of destroying bacteria and unwanted foreign matter, white blood cells called by such interesting names as polymorpholeucocytes, phagocytes, B-cells and T-cells. Kupfer cells, lining the spaces of the liver, consume bacteria from the blood as it is filtered. The cells of the Peyer's patches, in the small intestine, operate in a similar way, preventing destructive bacteria from attacking the intestinal wall. Special cells in the spleen destroy old blood cells.

The lymphatic system has thousands of miles of lymph vessels in the body, paralleling the blood circulatory system. Along these lymph vessels are found nodes ranging in size from a pinhead to a pencil eraser, and clusters of these nodes are found in the groin, armpits and neck. Lymph nodes filter out bacteria and foreign matter from the liquids of the body.

Specialized white blood cells circulate in the blood and lymph, destroying undesirable germlife and toxic waste as they go along.

Antibodies and a chemical substance called interferon work together to protect the body against viruses. Interferon is a chemical secreted in response to viral invasion, which protects cells and slows viral action. Antibodies are proteins whose job is to identify and destroy harmful viruses. In a complex series of actions, special cells first learn to identify the "weak spots" of harmful viruses, and then antibodies are manufactured which are able to track down these viruses, attach themselves directly to them, and destroy them.

When the elimination channels are underactive, toxic materials enter the blood and lymph systems too rapidly to be cleaned out by the liver and immune system functions. These toxic materials settle in the inherently weak organs and tissues, either directly causing under-activity, or inviting infection by viruses or bacteria. The immune system becomes increasingly underactive, leaving the body more and more unprotected against germlife, toxic wastes, and various chronic and degenerative diseases.

The strongest natural defense against disease is a clean, rested body, chemically balanced with the proper foods, with healthy, active elimination channels.

Chapter 9

CASE HISTORIES AND TESTIMONIALS

DISCUSSION BETWEEN DR. R., AN EMINENT OSTEOPATHIC PHYSICIAN OF ENTON HALL, ENGLAND, AND DR. BERNARD JENSEN, ABOUT THE TISSUE CLEANSING PROGRAM

Dr. J.   Doctor, you have just seen me go through a colema treatment. You have observed how the treatment works. Tell me what you think of it.

Dr. R.   To me, it is an eye opener and a verification of what I have believed and have tried to overcome in our own colonic machines; but I've never seen anything to equal the results that you are getting. I always felt it took weeks, if not months, of fasting and colonics to accomplish what you are getting in a relatively short length of time.

Dr. J.   Do you think the colema process is thorough enough to provide long-term benefits for the whole body?

Dr. R.   I am sure of it. Furthermore, when you are fasting, cleansing and eliminating, nature is squeezing her sponge. She is throwing these toxins into the intestinal tract, and you are able to bring them out in this spectacular way.

Dr. J.   Have you ever seen specimens from the bowel demonstrated as well as in this cleansing program?

Dr. R.   Never. In all my 50 year's experience with colonics, I've never seen anything to equal this.

Dr. J.   From my experience with the tissue cleansing program, I can't help feeling it is a process that would help everybody. I think many people would profit from a good cleansing that would help keep them from trouble like hardening of the arteries, cholesterol deposits, high triglycerides and so forth.

Dr. R.   This is preventive medicine at its best, because a toxic bowel is the sewer of the body. It is the most important eliminative structure of the system, and to get this cleansed out and to give it a chance to function normally, I think is fundamental.

Dr. J.   We have to compensate for the junk we've put into our bodies. I think it is almost a sin to have coffee and donuts, but God only knows I was raised on them. I grew up on Danish pastry. There must be something built into my body pattern that is still there to a certain extent, and I think that has to be cleaned out. This is one of those ways of going back and clearing out those toxins from polluted air, polluted water, junk foods and body acids induced by stress. To me, this seems the best way to compensate for all of that.

Dr. R.   Let's put it this way, it is the fastest and best way I know of.

Dr. J.   Don't you feel that this along with nutrition provides the fundamentals to start with?

Dr. R.   Absolutely. Clean out, and then build upon a sound nutritional basis. Most people only come to think seriously of these problems through personal ill health and not being able to find the solution. Then we start searching. Thank God, I landed in a naturopathic school.

Dr. J.   Well, I think it was a godsend that brought you here today to see this at the age of 78, after practicing 50 years. I am in the same position, up in the 70s, and now I see something that I didn't see before. Why wasn't somebody there to tell me? Don't you feel that same thing about this cleansing program?

Dr. R.   I am convinced of it. It's an eye opener. It gives you a new dimension to your thinking, a realization that bowel function and bowel toxemia are very real and very constant problems.

Dr. J.   Have you *ever* seen anything like this before?

Dr. R.   Never!

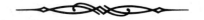

CASE HISTORIES

PATIENT 1

Patient complained of leg and foot problems; ulcers (open, running and partially encrusted on heel, instep and outside ankle of right foot; heel and instep of left foot); swollen ankles. The leg problems began two years prior to time of examination. Conditions previously treated without success by several physicians. Ulcers worsened. Unable to wear shoes for over a year. Unable to wear stockings previous three weeks due to increasing number of eruptions from ulcers. Blood pressure 80/58. Patient complained of cold hands and feet.

HISTORY. Severe diarrhea for previous seven and a half years. Seven or eight bowel movements per day. No relief from either drugstore medications or prescription drugs. Hospitalized with kidney stone attack in January 1976 (four years ago) with surgery recommended by hospital staff physicians. Refused surgery, treated self at wife's recommendation with vitamins and nutritional supplements for two months. No recurrence of kidney stone attacks since that time. (Lab test after examination showed creatinine level at 0.6 mg/dl—within normal range.) Family history of foot problems. Paternal grandfather died of gangrene which first appeared on right foot. Physician's diagnosis of grandfather included hardening of arteries, low blood pressure and diabetes. After right leg amputation, gangrene appeared on left foot. Amputation of left leg followed by recurrence of gangrene on stumps of both legs. Death resulted two years after left leg amputation. Patient's mother suffered from swollen right ankle during heat of summers in Midwest. Physician advised that problem was due to heart condition. Patient reported that his brothers and sisters all had varicose veins, as well as his paternal grandfather. Mother and one brother died of colitis. One physician who saw patient (an acupuncturist) diagnosed problem with feet as due to colitis, reasoning that male children inherit mother's problems, female children inherit father's problems. Patient left without taking treatments because the physician simply assumed the diagnosis. In 1976, patient had complete medical examination with EKG, chest X-ray, usual lab tests and several biopsies of the stomach. Medical report was negative for cancer. Nothing was found wrong except kidney stones, for which patient came in. Patient stated he had always had circulation problems.

IRIDOLOGY ANALYSIS. Black in intestinal area indicated underactive bowel with heavy toxic settlement there. Inherent weakness in kidney areas of irides. Adrenal glands underactive, showing that kidneys and adrenals were overworked due to toxic condition of blood from underactive bowel. Leg areas underactive. Poor circulation and enervation, together with underactivity in legs, indicated toxic settlements in leg tissues.

PROGRAM. Initially, Patient eliminated fried foods from his diet, reduced meat intake, increased raw salads and added several nutritional supplements. He reported, "The bowel has improved considerably...with bowel movements reduced from seven or eight per day down to twice a day. The feet, unfortunately, got worse." Patient was then placed on a seven-day tissue cleansing program which included two colemas per day, morning and night. (Colemas are not as strenuous as colonics but are more effective than enemas.) Fasting diet included broth, herb teas, vitamins, nutritional supplements and juice mixed with bulk and clay water. Clay packs and aloe vera were applied externally to the legs. On the fourth day, Patient reported, "The swelling in my right ankle is gone. It is now normal. The scaling or encrustations on my feet, ankles, insteps and heels, began to fall away. I would say there is a 60-70 percent improvement. I am elated over the results." Examination at this time showed strong improvement of ulcerated areas around feet. Patient is using skin brushing and cold water packs on body. Goal was to increase circulation and life force. Dulse was used to quicken the thryoid, and Dren-C was used to improve circulation. Pancreas substance was taken to dissolve the heavy mucus lining in the bowel. The elimination of mucus from the bowel was an important step toward improved assimilation of nutrients from food after end of tissue cleansing program. When the seven-day program had ended, Patient's feet had cleared up almost entirely. Ulcers no longer draining. Skin healing, becoming clear. Patient had worked very hard, cooperating with the program entirely. When asked for his response to the results of the seven-day tissue cleansing program, Patient reported, "It is almost miraculous! My wife and family are going to find it difficult to believe what they see when they arrive."

Patient was advised concerning the necessity of changing former food and other life habits to an improved nutritional and exercise regimen, to bring about general upgrading of health and to avoid recurrence of ulcerated leg problem. He was told that he had a year's work ahead of him. Although the ankles were now normal at the beginning of each day, swelling continued to occur around 11 a.m. or noon, particularly in the right foot. On the day patient returned home, he was able to wear shoes comfortably for the first time in over a year!

PATIENT 2

Patient's complaints were psoriasis, diabetes and arthritis.

HISTORY. Patient developed psoriasis 7 years ago. First symptoms were scaling of scalp and of facial skin under beard. Condition became progressively worse until 3 years ago, when fingernails began showing pits and creases. A year later, Patient developed diabetes and began taking insulin. Six months after the appearance of the diabetes, arthritis set in. First symptoms were fluid in the knee and inflammation of the elbow. A physician diagnosed the condition as psoriatric arthritis. Patient found that Western medicine could do nothing for his condition. He was taking 20 aspirin per day for relief from arthritic pain, insulin shots for the diabetes and the psoriasis was growing worse. He began to experience depression and hopelessness.

IRIS ANALYSIS. Inherent weaknesses in bowel and bronchials. Catarrhal congestion in lungs. Lymphatic rosary. Kidney weakness. Nerve rings. Pancreas weakness. Toxic thyroid. Scurf rim. Drug deposits—iron, sulfur and iodine.

PROGRAM. Patient was placed on a seven-day tissue cleansing program. From monitoring blood sugar level, Patient found it necessary to reduce insulin requirement gradually from 18 units down to nothing by the fifth day when blood sugar level remained within normal limits (70-110) without insulin.

RESULTS. Arthritis improved dramatically. Patient had difficulty putting on socks before but can now do that without problems. Walking was painful and is now normal. The severity of the diabetes is reduced. Psoriasis has improved but will take time to get skin back to normal. Skin is moister than before. Psoriasis peels in larger areas; peelings come off easier and there is little bleeding. Patient is in excellent spirits, looking forward to bicycling when he returns home.

PATIENT 3

Subject has had cancer for the last eight years. This is a cancer of the breast. Surgery removed a lump and it was found to be very malilgnant. Mastectomy was advised. Patient refused any further surgery and searched for alternative treatments and cures. She first went to laetrille therapy. Soon afterwards was under the care of a natural hygienist for 5 years. She followed a very strict program during this time. Breast became harder and harder. At one point a lump appeared near the surface and ruptured leaving an open, bleeding unhealing sore.

Patient had taken Dr. Jensen's lectures and courses in the past and at these times was advised to control a calcium deficiency and metabolic imbalance. Her doctor back home consistently refused the calcium control stating that it would be fatal for her to do so. She was afraid to not follow his advice and did not adjust the calcium as recommended.

Patient has had over 300 colonic treatments during this time. She was advised by Broda Barnes to stabilize her thyroid activity as he felt it was out of balance. This could cause a calcium upset. At one point, X-rays were taken of the back, revealing it to be like that of an 18 year old. Patient's health deteriorated rapidly.

She was advised at this point of advanced bone cancer. Her pelvic bone looked like Swiss cheese. She was told that she had 2 weeks to live and to go to Hawaii for her last days.

Patient immediately started calcium treatments and looking after her calcium needs. By now the tumor had broken through causing unbearable pain. She was taken to a hospital and given morphine. Her condition warranted being put on a terminal list during this visit.

She left the hospital and went to New Mexico and underwent heat treatments. During her visit there she broke her leg. By now the cancer was a large, oozing, bloody, open sore and was beyond a surgical remedy.

During this period she gave her life over to the Lord and experienced a major turning point. She advises that holding any negative thought patterns or resentments is absolutely lethal to well-being. These things will cause death to approach and cannot be indulged in if recovery or healing is to take place.

She started to take Dr. Jensen's advice wholeheartedly at this time. Combined with new attitude and nutritional improvement, the tide was turned and the tumor started to recede and heal. She has since taken the 3-day cleansing treatment.

The tumor is gone and all signs of the cancer are gone also. Laboratory tests are negative. This woman is a very good patient in that she did not give up and was willing to work hard and change her attitudes about life.

PATIENT 4

Phone call came today from a colema patient telling me that approximately the first part of November 1980, she started wheezing and coughing; also experienced aching all over the body. These were some of the past problems coming back.

In August 1979, she had a bad cold with wheezing. October of the same year, had to go into hospital in New York with a chest cold; again in November, had to be hospitalized for the same trouble; got to the point she could not take care of child.

She came here in February 1980 for a cleansing treatment, has had second treatment and has followed the maintenance program.

When the past problem recurred, she stopped her solid foods and used only potato peeling broth and soup; during this time, she took two colemas a day. Within two days, she was feeling much better and is doing fine now.

"Tell the Doctor thank God for the Colema!"

PATIENT 5

The following is a letter received from patient B.F., who received colema treatment in April 1980. Here is her report:

"I am dropping this note to let you know that the Tissue Cleansing Regimen which I took the first week in April cleared up the cysts in the breast which had troubled me. I hope to see Dr. Jensen at the Nutrition Workshop that he is going to teach in New Lebanon, New York this summer from July 21-28.

I plan to drive over for the day and, if possible, have Dr. Jensen examine me. He had wanted to do so and he will be able to see the changes in me since I have been following the colema regimen.

PATIENT 6

I had a call the other day from a man—a personal friend of mine who has been assisting in the care of an elderly lady, probably around 70. For the past couple of years she has had arthritis and last year she had to have an operation to have the spleen removed. They couldn't control the blood count unless the spleen was taken out.

She got along fairly well after the operation but then her arthritis came back still more. She had extreme pains throughout the whole body to the place where she could not control it and she had to be taken into the hospital where they could not find anything wrong with her.

X-rays showed nothing. The pain was so extreme they went into the bowel and found an obstruction. When she died, they said she died of septic shock. This is not unusual because it follows the pattern that we see with so many people.

PATIENT 7

Phone call in October. This person started the tissue cleansing treatment in June, the June before 1980 and her problem was degenerative disease in the female organs, principally the uterus. She was advised to have a complete hysterectomy because of suspicions of a very serious degenerative nature.

Four months later this woman went for her Pap test and an elimination. They found everything normal. She has finally returned to work and is very thankful for what has happened.

PATIENT 8

Twenty-six-year-old mother of three diagnosed as having Multiple Sclerosis. She has not been given any hope of overcoming this disease from her doctor. They have offered her nothing, no dietetics, no nutritional counseling, and no encouragement. She has been told by her professional guides that she can't get well with any treatments. That she must accept her condition and live with it.

With nothing to lose from this prognosis, she has been working with our system and reports that her vitality is better, she feels better and her nerves are much better; she is digesting her food better and her bowels are better.

PATIENT 9

This lady has gone through the tissue cleansing treatment twice. She has had considerable problems dealing with the spine, neck, joints, abdominal disorders, digestive disturbances, lung disturbances, bronchial problems; going through the change of life.

The cleansing treatment was 11 months ago and the second was 7 weeks later, as we advised. Following that, she has been living a fairly good life from a food and mental standpoint; adjusting her job; trying to do as much as she can for herself; having more sunshine treatments during the summer; circulation treatments through Kneipp baths; and trying to readjust her life to such an extent that she built herself up to a healing crisis; that reversal process that we talk so much about.

The healing crisis came and she developed pains and aches especially where she had been operated on for a disk in the neck. Then the pain went to the shoulder and different parts of the body. The intestinal problem became a little bit unmanageable so she went on the tissue cleansing treatment again. We planned for 3 days due to the fact that most crises only last about 3 days and we thought that this would be enough, but she stayed on the program for the full 7 day period.

She has had greater eliminations from the bowel during her healing crisis than at any other time. This is a very important thing to consider and I would like to discuss this for a moment.

First of all, we find that disease is a result of catarrh, mucus and phlegm settling in various parts of the body; toxic materials that have been in our blood over a period of years that have developed the kind of shoulder; the kind of joint material that we have in our body now.

We are reversing this, we are using an evolved way of eating; we're going a better way from a health standpoint. The reversal process goes right out through the tissues when they are regenerated to get rid of the old and to allow the new to come in. In other words, we're not building a new disease, we're going backwards now and in going backwards, we call this the reversal method of cleansing; the reversal method of getting rid of any disease accumulation that may be in the body.

In this case, we find that the second elimination treatment, at the end of 7 weeks, did not discharge much mucus or catarrh from the bowel. In contrast, during this crisis it was unbelievable what the tissue cleansing treatment and the colemas have brought down from the bowel. There were mucus strings and other materials that were unbelievable. They were of such a copious nature that there were two quarts at a time of this mucus membrane. It was foul and gave up a lot of gas. She had to resort to an extra colema treatment in order to take care of this toxic material that had settled in the bowel. After the 6th day, we found that the colema became clear again. There is still an excessive amount of material coming from the bowel. The greatest amount of toxic material came possibly the 4th, 5th and 6th days. It is beginning to ease up now and it is time that she moves on to the transition diet and the regular eating program once again.

This case has been mentioned because it illustrates clearly that during the healing crisis it may become a necessity to go on the colema treatment once again. I will say that everyone who follows this treatment is going to have these healing crises develop. It will bring back the problems that you have had in the past, symptoms you had 10, 20, 30 years ago. It is at this time that the toxic material should be eliminated because the body has liquified the catarrh, liquified the mucus and it is getting to a running stage. At this time, you help it with the colema.

After this is over, you will find that it will take 3 to 5 days for a complete elimination to occur, after which you're ready to start a better life than you've had in many years.

The healing crisis can be a short one, it can be a little one, it doesn't have to take long. Anybody going through this tissue cleansing treatment will get a strong healing crisis.

I feel that people overcome their troubles a lot quicker through this reversal process that they would any other way. You make more progress with this program than with any way I know of other than through extreme fasting.

PATIENT 10

This man suffers from extreme flatulence and X-ray shows severe diverticula of the colon. He has had kidney operations to remove large stones, and has been told that there is a large mass in one kidney. He hasn't the will to live because of these troubles. Blood pressure was high (188/120), extreme digestive disturbances, heart attack, gout; taking drugs now. Does not smoke or drink alcohol. Barium enema shows number of diverticula has tripled in one year's time.

Iris examination reveals deep, dark and large lesions in colon areas. Kidney areas indicate extreme underactivity.

Doctors want to take out sections of the bowel and have no other remedy.

He came to us with these troubles. The seven-day treatment was started with the tissue cleansing regimen. Good things started to happen immediately. He was able to get the first decent night's sleep in years by the third day. Flatulence has been reduced markedly. Patient says he hasn't felt as good in years. He claims that he feels like he has been given a new chance at life and is very optimistic about staying on the program. The opportunity to reverse his degenerative processes has given him hope that was not available before.

PATIENT 11

After taking treatments several months ago, the stomach trouble has left and the digestion is now better.

We have not heard any bad results from cases taking the treatment.

PATIENT 12

Patient had hepatitis. Tests revealed an almost normal condition after one month of colema treatment. Chemistry panel showed alkaline phosphorous of 1760 (normal is 79 to 250 IUL) went to 82 during this treatment.

She used no drugs, just foods and tissue cleansing system.

Chapter 10

IN CONCLUSION

"Should the body sue the mind before a court judicature for damages, it would be found that the mind had been a ruinous tenant to its landlord."

Essays of Plutarch

I have devoted my life's energies to discovering the secrets of happy, healthy long life. Searching the world over for examples of these blessings has been quite an experience and I've learned a great deal.

During the 50 years of practice trying to help people be and stay well, I've come to one certain conclusion. That the number one symptom that exceeds all others considerably is bowel disturbance.

People in this society and culture are all suffering some kind of digestive or eliminative malfunction. It is epidemic in proportion.

Our food and lifestyle are slowly doing us in by undermining the health and vitality of our great people. Sickness and disease are claiming a greater and greater portion of our energy, time, money and emotions. We are becoming health poor and vitality bereft.

We have strayed from the right path and have been led into a dead end prematurely. This is unfortunate but not inescapable. By turning around and giving up the old; cleansing, rejuvenating and taking the higher path, we can once again enjoy the wonderful blessings of a healthy, vital life as the Creator intended us to have.

We must defy the life-robbing habits and foods by refusing to partake of them anymore. We must be willing to cut loose of the old and like a little child once again learn the new, better ways. Surgery and drugs merely delay and antagonize the problems, rarely ever reaching the source of our diseases. One operation leads to another. Drugs are given to alleviate symptoms and mask over a deeper and often chronic condition that goes undetected and uncared for until it is often too late to correct.

There is one sure way to deal with our health problems. That is God's way. When we follow nature, we can't lose. It's perfect and always works. It is beyond man's tampering and contains all the preconditions for long, healthy life.

It takes a long time to develop a chronic, degenerative disease, and it takes awhile to reverse such conditions. But it is possible if the individual can attune his or her self to the task and have faith and perseverence in the natural healing powers of the body.

I've worked in bowel management all my life. I've tried every natural method, product or technique known to man that would care for the bowel.

Of all these things I can say that fasting and alfalfa tablets have done the most good of all. Now I want to tell you that the Ultimate Tissue Cleansing System is the greatest thing I've ever known to detoxify the body and clean the bowel. This is a recent development; one we have been working on all our lives. Now it is here when we need it more than ever before.

I'm not saying it's a cure all, but that it is a very powerful beginning for a person who is working toward an eventual healing. Anything we can do to stop autointoxication is going to help slow down the disease process. The Ultimate Tissue Cleansing System is the best way I know of to accomplish this goal.

By stripping down the old, toxic mucus lining of the bowel, we remove the number one source of disease in the body. In addition, we open up the bowel to a more efficient means of waste elimination and nutrient absorption, both of which are essential to any lasting healing process. This is also the first step toward normalizing the bowel so that the friendly bacteria will return to keep the colon safe from putrefaction and further autointoxication.

Doctor's wishing to learn this work may inquire about classes being given. Likewise, patients are being taken upon review and inquiry.

Here is a short story you might enjoy about one of the longest lived men in Western history.

"Westminster Abbey was begun by King Lucius in A.D. 170. The vaults are crowded with illustrious dead whose monuments cover the walls of the vast church. One of the smallest slabs—more interesting than all the fine marbles to princes and poets—says:

'Thomas Parr of ye county of Salopp, born A.D. 1483. He lived in ye reigns of ten kings: Edward IV, Edward V, Richard III, Henry VII, Henry VIII, Edward VI, Mary, Elizabeth, James I, Charles I. Buried here November 15, 1635. Aged 152 years.'

Before Parr was interred in Westminster, his history was carefully investigated. The parish register of his native village proves he was baptized in 1483. Legal documents and court entries show that he inherited a small farm from his father in 1560, and that he took a wife three years later when eighty. He married again in 1605 at the age of one hundred and twenty-two. When over one hundred and thirty he pleaded guilty, in court, to the charge of being the father of an illegitimate child. He was a farmer all his lilfe. His great age attracted the notice of the King who invited him to the palace for a visit, as the King wished to investigate his exceptional longevity.

Parr's last days were spent in the palace. History says his perfect faculties and marvelous memory made him a matchless entertainer. No wonder—what reminiscences a man, who lived in ten reigns, must have had!

After Parr's death, Harvey, who discovered the circulation of the blood, made an autopsy, by order of King Charles, to find out why he lived so long. The great surgeon's report in Latin, still preserved, states that Parr died from acute indigestion brought on by indulgence in unaccustomed luxuries.

All of the old man's organs were in perfect condition and Harvey describes the colon as normal in position and in other respects like that of a child.

Modern microbiologists say that in this report Harvey unknowingly reveals the secret of Parr's long life, because his minute description of the intestines proves that the congenital, protective flora had not been lost."

Pandora's Box—What To Eat and Why
J. Oswold Empringham, 1936

Today is a new day. We no longer have to carry skeletons in our closets. We no longer have to function on 2nd grade information or even 12th grade information; we can choose what grade of consciousness we want to live in. The Muscular Dystrophy campaign phrase "Your Change is the Key to the Cure" has more portent than we realize.

I would like to hand people a pair of invisible scissors and ask "What is that to thee?" Use those invisible scissors, cut it off and be free. Loosen it, let it go. "He leadeth me beside the still waters..." Do you know where the stillness is? Get rid of the confusion and mental chatter that you've had in the past. Be still and know...take a little time out...find out who you are...go forward with a sign on your back that says "Under New Management!" Meet the new day with a refreshed spirit!

BIBLIOGRAPHY

American Cancer Society, cancer literature.

BioNutritional Products, P.O. Box 389, Harrison, NY 10528.

Blending Magic, Jensen, Bernard, D.C., Escondido, CA.

Bon Roy Enterprises, 2425 Old Alturas Rd., Redding, CA 96003.

Chronic Intestinal Toxemia and Its Treatment, Wiltsie, James, A.B., M.D., 1938.

Colema Boards, Inc., P.O. Box 229, Anderson, CA 96007.

Colon Hygiene, Kellogg, John Harvey, 1923.

Diet and Nutrition—A Holistic Approach, Ballentine, Rudolph, M.D., Himalayan International Institute, Honesdale, PA 1979.

Diverticular Disease of the Colon, Painter, Neil S., M.D., Keats.

Doctor/Patient Handbook, Jensen, Bernard, D.C., Escondido, CA.

Food Healing for Man, Jensen, Bernard, Ph.D., Escondido, CA.

Health Magic Through Chlorophyll from Living Plant Life, Jensen, Bernard, D.C., Escondido, CA.

Invisible Friends of the Body, Empringham, J.; Health Education Society.

Intestinal Gardening for the Prolongation of Youth, Empringham, J.; Health Education Society, Los Angeles, CA.

Intestinal Ills, Jamision, Alcinous B., M.D., published by Charles A Tyrrell, M.D., 1914.

Intestinal Management for Longer Happier Life, Stemmerman, W. H., M.D., 1928.

Irons, V. E., Inc., Natick, MA 01760.

Jennings Home Colonic Boards. P.O. Box 1495, Anderson, CA 96007.

Lectures on Colonic Therapy, Schellberg, Boto O., 1930.

Nature Has A Remedy, Jensen, Bernard, D.C., Escondido, CA.

Pandora's Box—What to Eat and Why, Empringham, J. Oswald, Health Education Society, Los Angeles, CA.

Science and Practice of Iridology, Jensen, Bernard, D.C., BiWorld Publishers, Inc., 1952.

Survive This Day, Jensen, Bernard, D.C.

Take Care Health Products, Box 538, 1755 Robson St., Vancouver, B.C., Canada V6G1C9

The Chemistry of Man, Jensen, Bernard, Ph.D., Escondido, CA.

The Encyclopedia of Digestive Disorders, Roberts, Frank, Capt. M.D., M.N.I.M.H.D.B-TR. 1957-1969.

The Essene Gospel of Peace, Szekely, Edmond Bordeaux, IBS INTERNACIONAL, COSTA RICA, Central America.

The Human Body, Clendening, Logan, M.D., Alfred A. Knopf, New York, 1973.

The Human Body and How It Works, Exeter Books, NY 1979.

Toxemia Explained, Tilden, J.H., M.D. 1926.

Ultimate Colonics, Eldon L Lowder, 7835 South 1300 East, Sandy, UT 84092

You Can Master Disease, Jensen, Bernard, D.C., Escondido, CA.

GLOSSARY OF TERMS

The following list of words and terms is often used in describing bowel conditions and management.

I have attempted to limit the use of technical vocabulary as much as possible so as to keep this discussion on a level that anyone can follow, regardless of education or training.

Adhesion. 1. A holding together of two structures which are normally separate by new tissue produced by inflammation or injury. 2. A fibrous band which holds parts together which are normally separated.

Anus. The outlet of the rectum lying in the fold between the nates or buttocks.

Autointoxication. A condition caused by poisonous substances produced within the body.

Catarrh. An inflammation of the mucus membranes.

Chyme. The mixture of partly digested food and digestive secretions found in the stomach and small intestine during digestion of a meal.

Colostrum. Secretion from the breast before the onset of true lactation two or three days after delivery. The secretion contains mainly serum and white blood corpuscles. So-called "first milk."

Constipation. Difficult defecation; infrequent defecation with passage of unduly hard and dry fecal material; sluggish action of the bowels.

Diarrhea. Frequent passage of watery bowel movements. It is a frequent symptom of gastrointestinal disturbances and is primarily the result of increased peristalsis.

Diverticulitis. Inflammation of a diverticulum or of diverticula in the intestinal tract, especially in the colon, causing stagnation of feces in little distended sacs of the colon (diverticula).

Diverticulum. A sac or pouch in the walls of a canal or organ.

Enema. Introduction of solutions into the rectum and colon. This is done to stimulate bowel activity and to cause emptying of the lower intestine.

Flaccid. Relaxed, flabby, having defective or absent muscular tone.

Flatulence. Gas in the stomach and intestines.

Flexion. The act of bending or condition of being bent in contrast to extension.

Haustra. The sacculated pouches of the colon.

Hemorrhoid. A mass of dilated, tortuous veins in the anorectum involving the venous plexuses of that area. There are two kinds: external, those involving veins distal to the anorectal lilne; internal, those involving veins proximal to the anorectal line.

Hernia. The protrusion or projection of an organ or a part of an organ through the walls of the cavity which normally contains it.

Hyper-. Prefix meaning above, excessive or beyond.

Hypo-. Prefix indicating less than, below or under.

Ileocecal Valve. Sphincter muscles which serve to close the ileum at the point where the small intestines open into the ascending colon. It prevents food material from reentering the small intestines.

Indican. Potassium salt of indoxylsulfate, found in sweat and urine, and formed when intestinal bacteria convert tryptophan to indole.

Indole. A solid, crystalline substance found in feces. It is the product of bacterial decomposition of tryptophan and is largely responsible for the odor of feces. In intestinal obstruction it is absorbed and eliminated in the urine in the form of indican.

Intestinal Flora. The bacteria present in the intestines. The chemical nature of the contents of the intestines varies considerably with respect to the portion of the tract being considered. At birth no bacteria are present in the intestines but are found there very shortly thereafter. Favorable bacteria may protect the body from invasion by unfavorable ones, which cannot thrive in an acid condition. Also, certain medicines, particularly antibiotics, may cause drastic alterations in the number and kinds of bacteria present.

Iridology. The science and practice revealing inflammation, where located and what stage it is manifesting. The iris reveals body constitution, inherent weaknesses, levels of health and the transistion that takes place in a person's body according to the way he lives.

Lacteal. 1. Pert. to milk. 2. An intestinal lymphatic that takes up chyme and passes it to the lymph circulation and, by way of, the thoracic duct, to the blood vascular system.

Lactobacillus Acidophilus. An organism which produces lactic acid by fermenting the sugars in milk. Found in milk, feces of infants fed by bottle, and adults. Also present in carious teeth and the saliva.

Lactobacillus Bulgaricus. The bacillus found in fermented milk. Milk fermented with this organism is known as Bulgarian milk.

Lactose. A disaccharide which on hydrolysis yields glucose and galactose. Bacteria can convert it into lactic and butyric acids, as in the souring of milk. The milk of mammals contains 4 to 7% lactose.

Laxative. A food or chemical substance which acts to loosen the bowels (i.e., facilitate passage of bowel contents at time of defecation), and, therefore, to prevent or treat constipation. Laxatives may act by increasing peristalsis by irritating the intestinal mucosa, lubricating the intestinal walls, softening the bowel contents by increasing the amount of water in the intestines, and increasing the bulk of the bowel contents.

Lymph. An alkaline fluid found in the lymphatic vessels and the cisterna chyli. It is usually a clear, transparent, colorless fluid; however, in vessels draining the intestines it may appear milky owing to presence of absorbed fats.

Lymphocyte. Lymph cell or white blood corpuscle without cytoplasmic granules. They normally number from 20 to 50% of total white cells.

Mucilaginous. Resembling mucilage; slimy, sticky.

Mucosa. Mucous membrane.

Mucus or Mucous. A viscid fluid secreted by mucous membranes and glands, consisting of mucin, leukocytes, inorganic salts, water and epithelial cells.

Peristalsis. A progressive wave-like movement that occurs involuntarily in hollow tubes of the body, esp. the alimentary canal. It is characteristic of tubes possessing longitudinal and circular layers of smooth muscle fibers.

Peyer's Patch. An aggregation of solitary nodules or groups of lymph nodules found chiefly in the ileum near its junction with the colon. In typhoid fever, they undergo hyperplasia and often become ulcerated. Also called aggregated or agminated nodules or follicles.

Phlegm. Thick mucus esp. that from the respiratory passages.

Prolapsus. A falling or downward displacement of some part of the body, as the colon.

Protomorphogen. Cellular nuclear material extracted from specific animal tissues containing the essential building blueprint for the construction of that tissue. (Example: adrenal, thyroid, pancreas, etc., substances.)

Pyloric. Pertaining to the opening between the stomach and duodenum.

Rectum. Lower part of large intestine, about 5 in. (12.7 cm) long, between sigmoid flexure and the anal canal.

Spasm. An involuntary sudden movement or convulsive muscular contraction.

Spastic. Resembling or of the nature of spasms or convulsions.

Stasis. Stagnation of normal flow or fluids, as of the blood, urine, or of the intestional mechanism.

ADDENDUM

SURGEON LECTURES ON BOWEL IMPORTANCE

Not only are many bowel problems and surgeries avoidable through proper nutrition, but chronic diseases originating in the bowel can be prevented by a correct diet. Dr. Denis P. Burkitt, a famous English surgeon, told a group of 200 prominent U.S. physicians that problems like obesity, diabetes, hiatus hernia, appendicitis, diverticulosis, colitis, polyps and cancer of the colon are virtually unheard of among rural East Africans.

The rural East African diet is high in fresh fruit, vegetables and coarse-ground cereal grains. The rough bran from the grain absorbs water, increases the bulk of bowel wastes and speeds up elimination time, keeping the bowel clean and healthy. Conspicuously absent in the rural diet are white flour, white sugar and other refined carbohydrates so common in Western countries and urban areas of Africa. Burkitt's conclusions are based on data gathered in the Congo, Kenya, Uganda, Sudan and other underdeveloped parts of the world.

Evidence from cancer studies at the University of San Francisco indicates that a toxic colon and constipation are linked to the appearance of abnormal cells elsewhere in the body. Proper bowel care, according to Dr. Burkitt, through right nutrition is the key to preventing much disease and needless surgery. Overconsumption of refined carbohydrates, it is believed, is responsible for arteriosclerosis and diabetes, while absence of sufficient fiber content allows increased pressure changes in the bowel which lead to colon diseases. Excessive refined carbohydrates favor the growth of putrefactive bacteria in the bowel, alter bowel chemistry and invite ulcerative colitis, polyps and colon cancer.

Dr. Burkitt apparently believes that low builk in the diet and the excess intake of white sugar and white flour products contributes to or causes many of civilization's diseases. Bowel transit time for a Bantu native is more than twice as fast as that of the average Englishman, according to Dr. Burkitt's research. The length of time food wastes remain in the bowel determines how putrefactive they get, how much the undersirable bacteria multiply, how much fat is absorbed through the bowel wall and what sort of chemical toxins develop in and pass through the bowel.

Dr. Burkitt pointed out that African natives who move to cities for work tend to change their diets and get more diseases. They eat more white sugar and flour, less fiber food, and the effects soon show up in the bowel and elsewhere. Sir Arbuthnot Lane, physician to the Royal Family in England earlier this century, also believed bowel conditions were related to diseases elsewhere in the body.

Lane was impressed by research he observed in the laboratory of Nobel prize winner Dr. Alexis Carrel at the Rockefeller Institute in 1911. Carrell was growing "live" tissue cultures on microscope slides, and as long as the living tissue was fed every day and the wastes were washed away, the tissue thrived. If the cell wastes were not washed away, the cells gradually deteriorated and eventually died within four days. Lane became convinced that much disease is caused by the body's response to its own toxic waste products, particularly in the bowel.

It is significant that surgeons and physicians are beginning to understand the importance of bowel care in the prevention of disease. We cannot have a healthy body without clean blood, and we cannot have clean blood unless we have a clean bowel with good tone to move wastes along promptly. A toxic bowel is the source of many health problems.

TESTIMONIES

NOTE: We have not treated nor do we claim to treat any disease in our tissue cleansing program. We claim only that it is an effective means of cleansing the bowel. The following testimonies have been voluntarily submitted by persons who have taken the 7-day cleansing program.

Patient Donald Bodeen, DC, Poughkeepsie, NY

All my life I have been plagued with a sluggish colon and the constipation which attends it. On occasion, severe pain would occur as spasms would come and go. I can't begin to relate to anyone the myriad of problems this has caused in my life. I feel it has directly, and perhaps even greater, indirectly, been associated with more mental and physical anguish than I care to recall.

Not until the colon cleansing program, as taught by Dr. Jensen in his book, TISSUE CLEANSING THROUGH BOWEL MANAGEMENT, was accomplished was relief and healing made possible for me. I could not have hoped or dreamed for anything better. It is now a part of my life, and has been incorporated into my daily practice in my chiropractic office.

Patient Gerona Alderin, Breast Lumps

For years, I have been cleansing by various methods. I've spent thousands of dollars on colonics, medications, vitamins, seeing a lot of doctors and nutritionists with very little results. It wasn't until I took my own health care into my own hands that recovery started to happen. I had gallstones and kidney stones and got rid of them without surgery. Last summer I discovered lumps on my breasts. January 13, 1982, was the most traumatic day in my entire life when my entire body broke out in an extremely itchy rash. Nothing alleviated it. I trembled inside and out, felt hot and cold, couldn't concentrate or meditate and had no energy. I knew I had to do more than I was already doing, which was a lot.

Each "expert" I spoke to advised another vitamin or supplement or something to "try." I had heard about Dr. Jensen's books, Tissue Cleansing Through Bowel Management and The Doctor-Patient Handbook, and was doing a lot of reading on self-healing.

During the January 13 trauma, the only thing I could think to use was the lemon juice, cayenne pepper, maple syrup and water cleanse which I did for one week while I was scurrying around getting a colema board and making numerous phone calls to find out where to get the supplements for the cleanse. I had no one to advise me on anything as no one in my home area knew anything about it. Needless to say, I learned the hard way.

That 7-day fast was followed by a 7-day intensive cleanse, than the usual maintenance program advised by Dr. Jensen. I couldn't remember feeling so terrific for a long time. My energy was great, the color came back to my skin and my eyes started to turn blue again. Rest is advised during the cleanse but as I was self employed, I found those weeks to be the busiest weeks of my entire career. I had so much energy I just did not want to rest.

I do Latin-American and ballroom dancing and on those three Saturday evenings during the cleanse, I danced from 8 pm to 1 am nonstop. After the first week, I was asked if I had been to Florida as

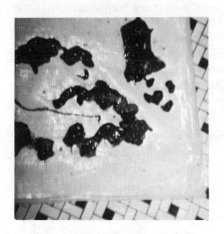

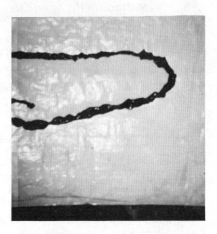

THESE PICTURES SENT IN BY ANOTHER PARTICIPANT.

ON THE 6TH DAY OF THE FOURTH CLEANSING, THERE WAS A 28-INCH LONG STRING OF MUCUS AND DEBRIS PASSED FROM THE BOWEL.

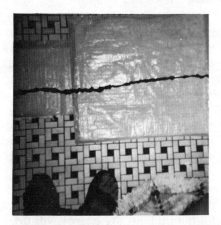

HERE IS ANOTHER PICTURE FROM THE SAME PATIENT ON ANOTHER DAY OF CLEANSE: 30-INCH-LONG MUCUS STRING PASSED.

My doctors are absolutely amazed and thrilled with my recovery, especially getting rid of the lumps on my breasts. I am seeing a chiropractor now instead of the numerous doctors I was seeing before. They are all telling me I am doing so well with this method that I don't need more appointments.

people said I looked so rested and had such good color. When I told my friends what I was doing, most panicked and were full of good advise as to what I should or should not do. They said it wasn't good for me to go without food; I would get too weak; I would get too thin; and I was even told I would die. They had to admit that I looked terrific, but still the pressure came forward. I had to be really strong and know that I was doing the right thing.

I have done six intense cleanses (Jensen's method) since January 1982. When I start to feel lethargic and ache all over, I know I have another build up of toxins. I get bored of doing the cleanse (taking the supplements mostly) after the 6th day and want to stop, but when I see what I am expelling, I am motivated to continue.

If I can get rid of lumps on my breasts, restore the color of my eyes to blue, have great skin color and tone, abundant energy and generally feel great, anyone can.

Patient M.T., Male, Degenerative Bowel Condition

I began the tissue cleansing treatments on September 8, 1982, and have continued with one colema every day since that time. I have had a degenerative bowel condition for some time, and the most spectacular result of the tissue cleansing has been the unbelievable material I have passed from my bowel.

Patient R.D., Male, Psoriasis

Since 1971, I had has psoriasis of the head area. On the fourth day of my tissue cleansing program, about 80% of the scales came off. This has never happened to me before.

I was happy to have a small healing crisis during the 7-day tissue cleansing program at Dr. Jensen's Ranch. When the fever, headache and eye aches began, I took a colema and passed much mucus and rubbery material. I felt much better, but later it returned. Another colema was taken, and this time about one or two quarts of rubbery fecal material passed out, leaving me free of symptoms. That night I passed mucus from my eyes, with a slight eyeache, but no fever or headache.

Patient A.M.B., Female, Rheumatoid Arthritis

When I began the tissue cleansing program, I could hardly use my hands. My left knee was so swollen I couldn't move it. During the program, my hands became more flexible, and the swelling and soreness in the palm of my right hand improved. The swelling in my knee decreased until I could walk without pain. My back is not aching all the time now and seems stronger. My feet aren't so tender on the bottoms.

Patient V.P., Male, Heart Condition

Before I took the tissue cleansing program, I had had a stroke, and my left arm was paralyzed. I arrived at the Ranch in a car driven by my wife. I was sitting in a reclining position from which I couldn't get up without severe stomach pain, and my face was pulling on one side as if stretching my mouth up. Only a few days before, I would wake up in the morning upset because life just didn't seem worth facing.

In four days I was able to climb into the shower by myself, put myself on the colema board and get off unassisted. I was able to get around without my cane.

I began to wake up happy in the mornings, able to get up from a reclining position without pain. My legs seemed smaller, not as much swelling. It was hard for me to believe the stuff that was coming out of me during the colema. Toward the end of the program, I seemed to develop a little feeling in my paralyzed left arm.

At the hospitals and nursing home, I never felt better, but during the tissue cleansing program at the Ranch, I continued to improve steadily.

Patient M.S., Female, Degenerative Lymph Condition

Three years ago I was told that I had a dangerous lymph condition which was treated and went into remission. I was very thankful but disappointed from the fact that although the condition had gone into remission, the cause was never explained, nor was it treated, but merely the symptoms.

A short while after this I happened to hear about Dr. Jensen's tissue cleansing program. I read his book on the subject and, in my opinion, everything made sense. I went on the program in December 1982. The elimination was unbelievable during my first 7-day cleanse. I have since been on two more 7-day cleanses using the maintenance program in between each. The results were amazing! I no longer felt lumps under my arms or in my groin. My breathing was clearer. I felt as if my whole body was becoming unclogged. My eyes became brighter and my skin softer and smoother. The veins in my legs are disappearing. I very rarely have depression as before. My hair and nails are in the best condition ever. I know I will never get any degenerative disease again as long as I eat the proper foods and keep my colon clean!

Patient H.E., Female, Scleroderma

I was diagnosed as having scleroderma in 1972 by a doctor who surgically removed a large calcified lump near my elbow. Scleroderma is a progressive skin disease often involving the internal organs such as heart and kidneys. I had a thickening of the skin and underlying tissue, great sensitivity to cold, a raw throat, dryness of lips and mouth, shortness of breath, fatigue and vague joint and muscle aches. In 1974, a doctor prescribed Potaba capsules, and this, in conjunction with biweekly chiropractic treatments, was effective in softening the skin and reducing muscle spasms.

On April 17, 1982, I started Dr. Jensen's 7-day cleansing program. By the end of the week, I noticed my skin was softer, the swelling had reduced in my hands and fingers and the red areas on my legs had faded. On the follow-up maintenance program, I found my mental outlook improved and I had increased tolerance to cold weather.

Patient S.D., Female, Anemia

When I started the tissue cleansing program, my lab blood test showed a red blood cell count of 3.84 (normal is 4.8) and a hemoglobin of 10.7 (normal is 14.0). I had been tired much of the time for the past several months and had lower back and neck pains. Chiropractic treatments didn't help. At the end of the 7-day program, my back felt much better, and I began taking supplements recommended by Dr. Jensen. A month afer my first blood test, a second blood test showed my red blood count was up to 4.47 and my hemaglobin was 12.8. My energy is much better, and the fatigue is gradually leaving.

Patient E.P., 70-year-old Female, Arthritis

The doctor who treated me said that drugs would bring the only relief for the terrible pains in my neck. So I took Percodan and Bulazolidin for pain; Phenylbutazone, a steroid, once a week and Ascriptin daily. I was told to eat anything I wanted, that coffee and diet had nothing to do with arthritis. I took these prescriptions for one year and still was not getting much relief.

Then I changed direction. I started a nutritional program, an elimination program and natural food supplements. I was asked to drop all drugs, much to my reluctance. I started trembling, and withdrawal symptoms developed. Nevertheless, I went right into the program outlined by Dr. Jensen.

Within a week, I found myself free of pain and feeling very well without drugs. One-and-a-half months later, feeling exceptionally good, I suddenly developed a fever of 105 degrees, swollen face and eye, with a headache such as I had never experienced before. I thought my whole world would collapse.

I was told it (the healing crisis) would only last 3 days—and it did! Then I felt so good again, just as Dr. Jensen said I would.

During and since the crisis, there has been excessive elimination of mucus. After nine months, my neck is still pain free without the use of drugs.

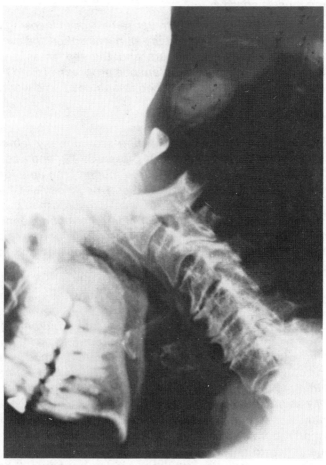

This is this patient's X-ray showing the arthritic condition.

After 5 years, she has no return of pain. This case has not been cured, but there has been no return of pain. This patient was taking 20-40 aspirin per day, according to her doctor's prescription.

Patient, S.B., Female, High Triglycerides

The first time I took the tissue cleansing program, my laboratory blood test showed a triglyceride reading of 938 (normal is 50-200 mg/dL). In a week's time, it dropped to 253. Nearly three years later, after a year of living under high-stress conditions, my triglycerides shot up to 1403 mg/dL. I went through the tissue cleansing again and the level dropped to 325. I realize there is more work to do, but I am delighted with the rapid drop of triglycerides following the 7-day programs.

NOTE: The triglyceride count and how they were reduced in this patient in just one week's tissue cleansing treatment.

BEFORE

AFTER

Patient, C.M., Female, High Triglycerides, 80 years old

Arthritic, bowel disturbances and gas, one movement every 4-5 days.

The pictures show what the before and after triglyceride counts, from medical laboratory tests, were for this patient. The changes were made in one week's tissue cleansing treatments.

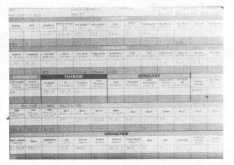

Triglyceride 50-200 mg/dL	Cholesterol 150-300 mg/dL
2544	633

BEFORE	ENLARGEMENT

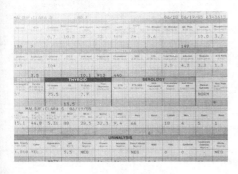

Triglyceride 50-200 mg/dL	Cholesterol 150-300 mg/dL
912	440

AFTER	ENLARGEMENT

Patient, C.B., Male

This is a swelling, edemous condition of the abdomen. He was an alcohol drinker and developed liver congestion. Medical doctors were unable to do much in elevating this over the last year.

The before and after pictures shown here were taken after just 30 days of treatment. The after picture shows him giving me a box of peaches weighing 28 pounds, and he said, "This is what you took off me in 30 days!"

This case is to show the value of the tissue cleansing program and what it can actually do. This is a demonstration of replacing new tissue for the old. The body responds to natural means of tissue replacement and follow-up on a good program of proper nutrition and lifestyle.

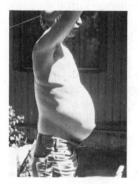

BEFORE   AFTER   AFTER

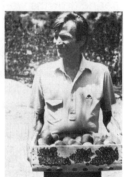

April 22 1988

Dear Doctor Jensen.

I was at your ranch in Escondido in 1984, the month of June I believe. I was there for a week and had a liquid retention problem. I have followed your recommendations as closely as possible ever since and consider myself to be in good health. I know that if I had not met you I would most likely have passed away a long time ago. I don't know how to thank you. My best wishes to you and Silvia.

Love

Christopher T. Bateman

Other Cases

Male, Prostrate Trouble. Lost 12 pounds on his first 7-day cleanse, prostrate problems cleared up, stiffness in hands disappeared. Can play musical instruments again.

Female, Constipation. Did not have bowel movement for 12-14 days, despite use of laxatives. After 7-day program, she stopped using laxatives, felt great. Bowel activity improving rapidly.

Female, Breast Lumps. One-and-one-half months after taking the tissue cleansing program, the breast lumps were gone. Also, lab tests showed liver function and alkaline phosphates were normal.

Female, Uterine Condition. A Paps test reading of 4+ and diagnosis of uterine growths were made before the 7-day cleansing. Three months after the program, a repeat Paps test and examination showed the condition was gone. The Paps test was negative, and no sign of uterine growths could be found.

Male, Psoriasis. This man had spent $7,000 on specialists, going to doctors all his life for psoriasis, before trying tissue cleansing. Arms and legs bleed periodically, and he has been a heavy drinker of alcoholic beverages. He has not taken the full 7-day cleanse program, but has been using the bulk and Bentonite and colema board. Skin condition has improved considerably.

Female, Memory and Vision Problems, 60 years of age. This elderly vegetarian woman complained of poor memory and poor vision. She took the 7-day cleanse and was astonished at the improvement in both.

Female, Uterine Fissure, 32 years old. Patient reported great pain for years from a uterine fissure, with no help from doctors. She took the 7-day cleanse as a last resort, but stopped at 5 days. She reported, "The pain all disappeared. I can't remember when I was last free of pain. I had forgotten what is was like."

Some comments from patients who have taken the tissue cleansing program.

"I can't imagine any better way to detoxify the body."   A.C.

"I think everyone should have the good fortune to go through this program so that they will know what really being alive feels like."   E.B.C.

"A tremendous value to humanity."   M.S.

"A wonderful start for your recuperation." E.N.

"Very necessary for renewed health." E.A.

"Great!!! Lovely staff also." P.M.

"After the week's program I felt hopeful! and excited about the potential for healing. I have learned so much." A.M.

"I liked the program very much as I felt better as the days went by." C.C.

"A positive and realistic program." O.S.

"Very good, wished I had done it sooner, would recommend it to anyone." J.E.W.

"Reasonable solution to good health." M.K.M.

"This is imperative for nearly everyone I know. Having studied a lot along this line, I feel it is as simplified as can be and still be effective. I shall never forget this time in my life." R.A.

"I feel more positive and hopeful. That I will learn what is missing in my diet and will follow through." C.M.

"After this program I feel energized! My body feels good, ready to go." S.M.

"I felt light and feel like exercising. I feel like a new person with hope in my heart." M.P.

"I feel light, optimistic, energetic. I'm looking forward to continuing on this program." L.D.

"I feel wonderful! Lighter and more energized than ever! On the road to greater health." W.J.R.

"(Before the program) I felt very tired, morose (that's not quite depressed) and a little caged in, because I didn't know how to properly handle the healthy aspects of life. (After the week's program) I was more than pleased with the program. It's excellent!" D.D.H.

"Before the program, I felt tired; had problems walking; pain. After the program I had less swelling; walked better; less joint pain. This wonderful program is lifesaving. I met many wonderful people. Many thanks to everyone for support." K.M.

"Before the program I had a definite need to learn bowel management, cleansing of tissue, etc. I know I need to improve my health or suffer consequences very rapidly. I felt very toxic; had memory

loss and pain in the head. Pain in right side near ribs. Terrible broken veins in legs. Tired much of the time and would depend on coffee to stimulate. After the program I felt much better, There is still room for improvement, but I feel very encouraged. The program is terrific. There should be more programs throughout the States." M.F.W.

"I attended the program after reading the book. Thought the treatment might help with various symptoms (sore breasts, fibrocistic), water retention, low energy, easy weight gain and some joint discomfort and neck kinks occasionally and occasional headaches. All of these symptoms affected my disposition and attitude. After the program I felt better! The breasts are softer, a bit less sore; abdomen smaller; energy still low; water retention still evident; didn't lose much weight." H.F.

"I attended the program because I was so tired; had leg and hip problems (limped); no one knew how to help. Doctors said I was healthy, but I knew I was not. I knew this program was right for me. After the program, I know how to care for me. I am very thankful for the privilege of attending. If I had not seen the filth expelled, I would never have believed it was in my body. I am looking forward to a healing crisis. The program is marvelous. People think I am out of my mind. Nevertheless, I am happy!" E.L.W.

A 78 year-old-man from Manitoba (Canada) phoned to ask if I would help him. I had previously helped some of his family members. He had been bedridden two years with ulcerated legs, the ulcers oozing pus. He was scheduled to have his legs amputated at the hips. I sent his daughter down with the equipment and supplements for the 7-day cleanse, and he was faithful, and redid it two weeks later.

The result was excellent. The last I heard of him, he was jacking up his garage to move it so he could have a bigger organic garden. It only took two weeks to get him mobile, and he's a happy man.

B.W.

British, Columbia
Canada
